the

fast diet

recipe book

the fast diet recipe book

MIMI SPENCER

WITH DR SARAH SCHENKER

PHOTOGRAPHY BY ROMAS FOORD

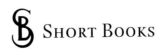

SHORT BOOKS

If you are on medication of any description, please see your doctor before embarking on any fast. There are certain groups for whom fasting is not advised. Type 1 diabetics are included in this list, along with anyone suffering from an eating disorder. If you are already extremely lean, do not fast. Children should never fast, so this is a plan for over-18s only. Pregnant women should eat according to government guidelines and not limit their daily calorie intake.

For more information and support, go to thefastdiet.co.uk

for debs

Published in 2013 by Short Books
3A Exmouth House
Pine Street
EC1R 0JH

10 9 8 7 6

Copyright © Mimi Spencer Ltd
Photography copyright © Romas Foord
Design: Georgia Vaux

Printed in Great Britain by Butler
Tanner & Dennis, Frome, Somerset

A CIP catalogue record for this book
is available from the British Library.

ISBN 978-1-78072-187-3

contents

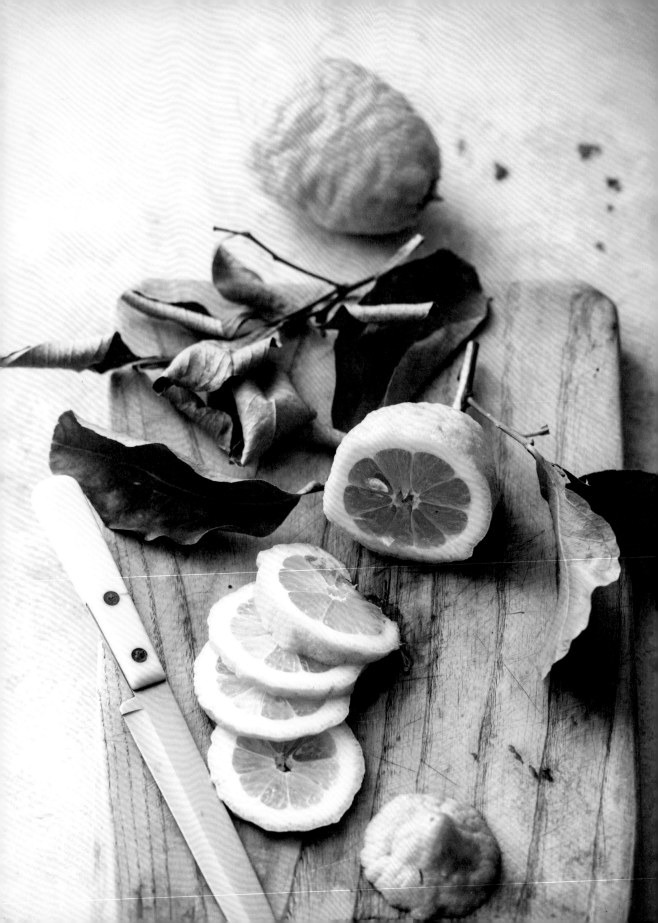

ALL YOU NEED TO KNOW ABOUT THE FAST DIET

How the Fast Diet went global

When Dr Michael Mosley and I started to sketch out plans for *The Fast Diet* book in October 2012, we had little idea that its impact and potential would prove to be so great. In the months since, the book has received a hugely positive response, and interest around the world is growing daily – from Korea, Brazil, Israel, Australia, the USA, anywhere where people are looking for a leaner, fitter life. Hundreds of people have written to us, often with great tenderness and emotion, about their weight loss and health improvements. There has been much enthusiasm from people in the public eye too. As food writer and cook Hugh Fearnley-Whittingstall wrote in the *Guardian*: 'I find myself beguiled, for the first time ever, really, by a new diet. *The Fast Diet*, by Michael Mosley and Mimi Spencer, makes a compelling promise that with regular fasting (they propose two days out of every seven) you will quickly lose weight... I believe in this fasting thing, I really do... I've lost eight pounds already, and I find the whole thing rather exhilarating. I feel I might just be part of a health revolution.'

Allison Pearson, in the *Daily Telegraph*, described *The Fast Diet* as her 'new bible': 'I no longer feel the need to sleep in the afternoon. My stomach has definitely shrunk. The other night it protested when I tried to finish dinner: a world first. Scientists swear that the fasting diet will add years to your life. Me, I'm just happy to have finally shifted that stubborn baby weight. About time, too. The baby was 17 last week.'

At thefastdiet.co.uk, the comments and questions keep rolling in. The Fast Diet has always been a conversation, never a set of commandments; we are not interested in promoting diet dependency, only in investigating an idea that appears to have significant health-giving potential. So, we're fascinated by your stories, your successes, your occasional blips, and as the science develops, we hope to have more answers to share.

In the meantime, many of you have requested inspiration for what to eat on your bi-weekly Fast Days. If you'll excuse the obvious oxymoron, this – *The Fast Diet Recipe Book* – is our answer. But before we pull on an apron and raid the fridge, it's worth having a brief detour into the science behind Intermittent Fasting, and how The Fast Diet came to be.

In the beginning...

In 2012 Dr Michael Mosley, an overweight, medically trained journalist, discovered that he was a borderline diabetic with very high levels of 'bad' cholesterol. He was told by his doctor that he needed to start medication and that unless he did something about it, within 10 years he would be swallowing eight pills a day, like the average 60-year-old European or American.

Keen to find a non-pharmaceutical way to change his fate, he tracked down and interviewed scientists engaged in cutting-edge research into Intermittent Fasting. 'Fasting', in this context, does not mean avoiding all food; it simply means cutting back, for relatively short periods of time, on some foods.

In our society, we tend to eat all the time – and that constant over-eating doesn't just make us fat, it also keeps our bodies in permanent 'go' mode. This leads to elevated levels of hormones like insulin and IGF-1 (insulin-like growth factor 1), which cause metabolic changes in the body. While these are a perfectly normal response to eating, the problem arises when they dominate all the time; this can bring an increased risk of developing a range of diseases including diabetes, heart disease and some cancers.

Cutting back on calories, by contrast, reduces insulin levels and gives your system a chance to rid itself of old and worn-out cells – a bit like taking your car into the garage for an occasional repair; doing so will almost certainly ensure that it goes on running in peak condition for longer.

The importance of fat loss versus weight loss

Weight is, of course, easy to measure – you just need bathroom scales. But what people sometimes forget in their obsession with 'losing weight' is that what they really want to lose is fat.

Not all fat, however, is equally bad. Fat on the thighs and buttocks appears to be less of a health risk than excess belly fat, known as visceral fat. Visceral fat significantly increases the risk of heart disease and diabetes, which is why you should aim to have a waist (as measured round your belly-button) that is less than half your height.

While losing fat, you want to preserve as much muscle as possible. One reason why it's important is that muscle is metabolically active; in other words, if you take two people who are the same weight, but one is muscular and the other fat, then the muscular one is not only likely to be healthier but will also burn more calories, even when sleeping. People with more muscle have a better chance of keeping weight off.

You can help preserve muscle by maintaining, or better still increasing, the amount you exercise. This could simply mean walking more and always taking the stairs, or more vigorous activities such as weight training. As an added bonus, studies have shown that you are likely to burn more fat if you exercise in the fasted than in the fed state.[1]

Intermittent Fasting and fat loss

One of the great problems with crash diets or 'yo-yo dieting' is that although some of the weight loss will be fat, much of it will be muscle (on a conventional diet you lose around 75% of weight as fat and 25% as muscle). When you regain the weight, as most people inevitably do, the weight you regain is almost all fat.

The human trials that have been done so far suggest that Intermittent Fasting is unusual in that the weight loss appears to be almost all fat, and, importantly, much of the fat you will lose is the dangerous type from around the gut.

A number of studies involving overweight volunteers doing ADF (Alternate Day Fasting)[2] found that when individuals were asked to eat a quarter of their normal calories one day, then eat whatever they liked the next, they lost significant amounts of weight and saw substantial improvements in their cholesterol and blood sugars. A surprising finding was that people, when allowed to feast, did not do so. They reported not feeling particularly hungry after a 'fast' day and rarely ate more than 110% of their normal calories. This is born out by anecdotal evidence too: many people on the Fast Diet simply don't feel ravenous the following day. Their appetite and attitude to food seems to change, and healthier eating seems to become part of their everyday life.

Another surprising finding was that on this form of IF, individuals lost more body fat than expected. In the most recent study of 32 volunteers followed for three months, the average weight loss was 4kg, almost all fat, and they lost an average of 3 inches around the waist. In another study, 107 women were randomly allocated either to a diet where they cut their food intake to 650 calories for two days a week and tried to stick to a healthy diet for the rest of the week, or to a diet where they consumed the same number of calories, but spread out over the week.[3] After six months, the two-day fasters had lost an average of 6kg of fat and 3 inches from their waists, compared with 4.9kg and 2 inches for the daily dieters. They also had much greater improvements in their cholesterol and insulin levels.

Enter the Fast Diet

So, there is evidence from human trials of success with different forms of Intermittent Fasting. Michael, after some self-experimenting, settled for a form he called 5:2, which is the basis of the Fast Diet. The rules are very simple:

- You eat normally for 5 days a week and then for 2 days a week you eat a quarter of your normal calorie intake — around 600 calories for men, 500 for women

- You can do your Fast Days back to back or split them. Michael tried both ways and found he preferred to split them. He did his Fast Days on Mondays and Thursdays

- He also split his 600-calorie allowance on those days into breakfast and an evening meal

On this regime Michael lost 19lb of body fat and his blood markers improved beyond recognition. He found that once he had lost the fat he could keep it off (normally the hard bit) by using the 6:1 method of cutting calories to a quarter of his normal intake once a week, and always taking the stairs.

Commissioned to write about Intermittent Fasting for *The Times*, I soon followed Michael's lead and in four months lost 20lb, returning to my 'wedding weight' at the age of 45. Towards the end of 2012, inspired by the success of the 5:2 pattern, Michael and I co-wrote *The Fast Diet* book. It became an instant bestseller, on both sides of the Atlantic. Intermittent Fasting really is, as Hugh Fearnley-Whittingstall says, starting to look like a 'health revolution'.

We believe that the Fast Diet's success has to do with its flexibility, its simple basic tenets, and the fact that it is backed by solid science. From a psychological point of view, its indisputable attraction is that calorie restriction is limited to 2 days a week, leaving the rest of the time blissfully free of worry.

So where's the catch?

There are some people for whom Intermittent Fasting is not recommended (see page 4), however, there is no evidence of significant side effects. Some people may experience headaches or constipation, particularly at first; these can generally be alleviated by drinking lots of calorie-free fluids and eating foods that are rich in fibre. Some find they get hungry late at night and can't sleep well. It should help if you have a more substantial evening meal, or perhaps a glass of milk before bedtime.

In some ways, the Fast Diet is simply a modern take on an ancient idea. Fasting, in one form or another, has been practised for centuries by most of the great religions, and if done properly seems to be extremely safe.

There are, however, a number of myths around eating that might dissuade you from trying Intermittent Fasting. These include the idea that:

- You need to eat whenever you feel hungry

- Eating every few hours will increase your metabolic rate

- If you don't eat every few hours your blood sugar will fall and you will feel faint

None of these widely held beliefs is backed by science. Certainly, fasting in any form can be tough to start with, but you should discover that short bouts of hunger are manageable and soon pass. Similarly, there is no metabolic advantage to spreading your calories over the day, nor is there any evidence that short periods without food will cause your blood glucose to plunge to seriously low levels. Most nights, you go 12 hours without eating and many people feel fine with a late breakfast.

You may want to get practical support before you start or if you have any queries. You will find a wealth of tips and supportive advice from those who have tried it at thefastdiet.co.uk, where you can also contribute your experiences. By now, though, you're probably feeling peckish. Time to move out of the classroom and into the kitchen.

Do you really want to cook on a Fast Day?

We're all different. When fasting, you may not wish to spend time in the kitchen, surrounded by ingredients and temptation. Some people want speed and simplicity, preferring to eat sparingly and basically — and there are plenty of ideas in this book that will be useful for this approach.

Others, like me, prefer to make Fast Day food interesting and flavourful, with fresh, low-calorie meals to book-end the day. I can't promise the glorious depth of glossy butter sauces, or the fudgy puds found in other cookbooks. There are no puds at all here. But I can offer wholesome, well-balanced, nutritious, engaging, pretty, fresh food that's simple to prepare and easy to understand. I will also suggest more unusual dishes to stretch the imagination and take us all on a bit of a journey.

A diet for foodies

In fact, I would even argue that the Fast Diet is 'a diet for foodies'. While you restrict calories — deliciously, if you wish, with as much fanfare as you dare within the calorie budget — on 2 days a week, the other 5 days you can eat absolutely normally. We don't suggest bingeing, but we do advise forgetting that you are on a diet at all. On 5 days a week, the Fast Diet is, and should be, an irrelevance.

What Intermittent Fasting *will* do, however, is encourage you to cut back on processed food, together with the attendant preservatives and packaging. It insists that you eat fresh, good produce for 2 days a week. The upshot? Over time? We are all more engaged with the food on our plates.

And the frugal

On the Fast Diet, you occasionally eat less, ergo you spend less, an idea well suited to these days of austerity. One Fast Diet fan, Snorvey, writes of his shopping bills: 'They're certainly lower. I hadn't even thought about it until someone mentioned it elsewhere, but at a rough guestimate, they're around 15% lower. A projected amount of 395,000 calories of food not eaten per annum (between two of us — the wife is following the 5:2 as well) would add up to a fair bit of money over the year.'

And non-fasters too

This book will help you develop a loose repertoire of meals that are sometimes hasty, always tasty, but above all low in fast-release carbs, which means that if you are calorie-counting in the traditional way — day in, day out — this book will serve you equally well: you could happily use it as an everyday low cal cookbook.

In fact, one of the key changes that will hopefully occur over several months on the Fast Diet, as many fasting fans have attested, is that your appetite will alter and you will start to crave the good things in life, *on any day*: you may develop a yen for fresh salads, fabulous soups, lean proteins, sparky flavour combinations, or satiating breakfasts that don't unduly bother the frying pan. You'll find countless recipes here that meet these requirements. The book works, too, for people who are dairy- or wheat-intolerant, as very few of the recipes contain either. And it's also pretty good for vegetarians, as lots of the recipes rely on plant proteins.

When you're not fasting, the book still has plenty to offer: play around with some of the ingredients, bump up the numbers, add a chunk of sourdough bread or a tumble of noodles, rice on the side or buttered corn-on-the-cob, and all of them will make for good eating on any day of the week.

WHAT, WHEN AND HOW TO EAT ON A FAST DAY

What to eat?

There are very few rules here. No weighing out 'matchbox-sized' portions of cheese. No measuring, fretting or complicated equations. In a nutshell, the Fast Day meal mantra is 'Mostly Plants and Protein'.

This is the basis of all of the recipes in this book. OK, there's a little fat too, a few slow-burn carbs, perhaps a drop of dairy. But 'Mostly P&P' pretty much sums it up. The only other word we'd add is variety. A varied plate of food promises a diverse line-up of nutrients and will add interest to your day.

So what should be on your Fast Day plate?

First, the question of carbs

One of the more important hormones determining your health is insulin. When you eat, particularly foods rich in carbohydrates, your blood glucose levels rise and in response the pancreas churns out insulin. Insulin helps to remove glucose from your blood and store it in your liver or muscles as glycogen. It also stops your body from using fat as a fuel.

If you constantly consume lots of sugary, carbohydrate-rich food (and drinks), your body copes by producing increasing amounts of insulin. In time, your cells become less responsive and your body is caught in a vicious cycle in which it has to produce ever-higher levels of insulin to get the same result. This can lead to type 2 diabetes, which in turn significantly increases your risk of heart attack, stroke, impotence, going blind and losing your extremities due to poor circulation. It is also associated with brain shrinkage and dementia.

An added problem is that as well as being a sugar- and fat-controller, insulin, together with the hormone IGF-1, stimulates the growth and turnover of new cells. This constant activity increases the risk that some of these cells will turn cancerous. High levels of insulin and IGF-1 are associated with a range of cancers including breast, bowel and prostate cancer.

There is good evidence that restricting your calorie intake, and in particular your carbohydrate intake, for a couple of days a week will improve insulin sensitivity and cut levels of circulating insulin. The recipes in this book are based on that approach, referencing the Glycaemic Index and Glycaemic Load of the ingredients. You'll recall that the GI rating measures the effect of a food on blood sugar relative to pure glucose (which scores 100). The GL takes into account how much of the carbohydrate is in the food. A watermelon, for example, has a high GI but a relatively low GL as it's mostly water.

On the days when you are fasting you still eat, but you should aim to eat foods with a low GI; in other words, foods that do not cause spikes in blood sugar. Most vegetables are a Fast Dieter's friend because they have a low GI, but also because they provide a lot of bulk for very few calories, keeping hunger at bay.

Protein

Protein, unlike fast-release carbohydrates, keeps you feeling full for longer, which is one reason to have plenty of it in Fast Day meals.

When people see the word 'protein' they generally think of meat. Though chicken and beef are rich in protein, there is also protein in fish, milk, nuts, seeds, pulses and legumes. Proteins are essential nutrients, the building blocks of your body tissue as well as a major fuel source. Unlike fat or carbohydrates, your body does not store protein; instead, food containing protein is broken down by your digestive system to provide amino acids, which are then used for a whole range of vital things, from building muscle to creating hormones, enzymes and neurotransmitters.

Because your body does not store protein, we recommend that you boost the protein content of your diet on Fast Days, so that it becomes a greater proportion of your daily diet on just those days. That way, you benefit from its satiating effects (protein really does make you feel fuller for longer than carbs) and you will have adequate levels of protein at all times. On non-fasting days, of course, we recommend that you eat as normal and don't concern yourself with dieting.

The recommended daily level for protein is roughly 55g per day. If you want to be more precise, one guideline suggests 0.83g per kg of body weight – which for a 70kg man would work out at about 58g a day, and for a 60kg woman around 50g.

Plants

The pigments that plants produce don't simply attract pollinating insects; they represent some of the thousands of bioactive compounds, known as phytochemicals, which keep plants alive and healthy. By eating a wide range of different-coloured plants we also get the benefits, and on a Fast Day, they are the central event.

Green
'Leafy greens', which include spinach, chard, lettuce and kale, are a good source of minerals like magnesium, manganese and potassium. Another class of green vegetables, the cruciferous ones, are those that contain sulphur and organosulphur compounds. These include cabbage, cauliflower, broccoli and other members of the brassica family. Sulphur is essential for the production of glutathione, an important

antioxidant, as well as amino acids such as methionine and taurine.

Different veg will bring different things to your plate: spinach, for example, contains lots of calcium, but it is not in a form that the body can readily absorb; if you want calcium, you are better off with broccoli. You can learn more from the 'Nutritional Bonus' included on each recipe page.

There are very few rules here. No weighing out 'matchbox-sized' portions of cheese. No measuring, fretting or complicated equations

---

Orange and yellow
Flavonoid comes from the Latin word *flavus*, meaning yellow, and in a plant this substance attracts insects for pollination and protects against harmful ultraviolet light. In humans there is some evidence that eating flavonoids helps combat the risks of allergy, inflammation and infection.[4] Fruit and vegetables with a significant amount of yellow or orange, such as carrots, melons, tomatoes, peppers and squash, contain a particular type of flavonoid called carotenoid. The type of carotenoid in carrots can be converted to retinol, an active form of vitamin A, important for healthy eyesight, bone growth and regulation of the immune system.

Red
There are a huge number of carotenoids, with different properties. Another class produces the colour red and is called lycopene. You'll find lots of lycopene in tomatoes. They are antioxidants and a recent study showed they help reduce the risk of having a stroke.[5] Oddly enough, cooking tomatoes boosts the levels of lycopene, because heat helps break down the plant's thick cell walls,

making the nutrient more available for absorption.[6] Unfortunately, heat also destroys vitamin C, so it's a trade-off.

Blue and purple
Blue and purple foods get their colour from a group of flavonoids called anthocyanins. You'll find decent levels in blackberries, blueberries, purple carrots and red cabbage. There is some evidence that anthocyanin-rich blueberries may slow the rate at which memory and cognitive function decline as people age.[7]

White
Examples include garlic, white onions, shallots and leeks, all rich in allyl-sulphur compounds. Although there is no compelling proof that garlic will ward off vampires, it does appear to be quite good at killing micro-organisms; traditionally, it was eaten raw to treat coughs, colds and croup.

Veggies: the raw and the cooked

There is debate about the best way to cook vegetables in order to retain as much of their goodness as possible. The answer is that there is no single answer. It all depends.

The reason we cook food is to make it more digestible; it tenderises meat, and breaks down tough vegetable fibre, something our digestive systems can no longer really cope with. But cooking also affects certain vitamins. Vitamin C, for example, is fragile and easily lost when heated, whereas lycopene is enhanced by the cooking process. If you live on a raw-food diet, it's likely that you will enjoy high levels of vitamin C, but low levels of lycopene. Boiling and steaming carrots, spinach and cabbage will also increase the bioavailability of carotene while reducing some other vitamin content. Our advice would be to mix up raw and cooked. Have both. Often.

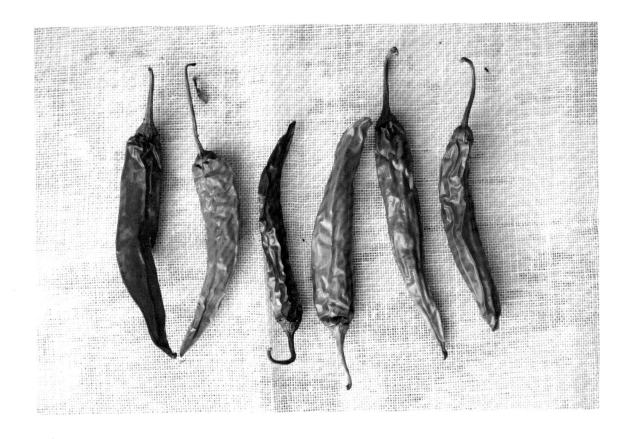

Why veg smashes fruit every time

When people are told they need to eat more fruit and vegetables they frequently respond by simply eating more fruit. On the face of it, that's no bad thing as fruit, like vegetables, is packed with nutritional goodies. Unfortunately, many fruits are also packed with calories and fructose. Vegetables, by contrast, provide a lot of bulk, masses of fibre and have limited impact on your blood sugars and therefore on your insulin.

Some fruits, like strawberries and blueberries, do have surprisingly few calories and do not adversely affect your blood sugars (unless, of course, you drench them in sugar), which is why you will find them in the recipes here. Blackcurrants and raspberries do respectably well too. Others, however, such as pineapple, are high in sugars. A large banana, for example, has around 120 calories, while a large carrot has about 30 calories and a large serving of broccoli about the same. So, while in general we would certainly encourage people to eat fruit, we recommend that sweet-tasting fruit should be rationed on a Fast Day.

If you do choose to eat fruit, make it fresh, not dried, as the drying process concentrates calories. A 100g serving of fresh apricots, for instance, typically has around 31 calories while the same quantity of dried apricots clocks up four times the calorie cost.

Many of these recipes work well as anytime meals. You may wish to skip breakfast, or dodge dinner. That is entirely up to you. The Fast Diet has been called the ultimate flexible diet with good reason

To juice or not to juice?

Although fruit is generally a nutritious option, juice is ultimately a higher-sugar, lower-nutrient version of its source. Juicing inevitably reduces or eliminates fruit and vegetable skin – yet those vital health-giving pigments, the seats of flavonoids and carotenoids, are concentrated in the skin (and, in some cases, the pulp). Your grandmother was right: eat the skin.

Plant skins are also the primary, if not the sole, source of fibre, important for the health of your gut – and also for slowing down the digestion and absorption of sugars. The take-home message is this: juice can offer a decent source of nutrients on days when it's hard to work in your usual amount of fruit and veg, but it's not an adequate substitute for the real, whole source.

Good fats and why you need them

Fat matters, and there is such a thing as too little fat in the diet. This is because certain vitamins (A, D, E and K) are fat-soluble, which means that they require fat in order to be absorbed by the body (B vitamins and vitamin C are water-soluble and don't need fat for absorption). Essentially, dietary fat ferries vitamins across the cell walls of the small intestine, into the bloodstream and on to the liver, where they are stored until the body needs them. But not all fats are equal. On a Fast Day, reduce saturated fats (animal fats), avoid trans fats, and instead choose plant fats, from nuts, seeds, olives or avocados. You only need a little, added to a vitamin-rich meal. The recipes in this book do just that, so you don't even have to do the sums.

Why soup?

You'll notice that there are plenty of recipes for soup in this book, and you may question their inclusion, given our advice on juicing fruit. Soups are a special case, and well worth including on a Fast Day menu. Research has shown that, while fluids generally have lower satiety value than solid foods, soups break the rule: they are brilliantly satiating, leading to what scientists at Indiana's Purdue University call 'reductions of hunger and increases of fullness... comparable to the solid foods'.[8,9] In short, soup gets you full and keeps you there. Great news for a Fast Day. Better yet, a home-made soup uses up elderly fridge veg, never tastes the same twice and will warm the cockles of your heart.

When to eat?

The timetable is largely your own. Eat when it suits you, your family, your lifestyle, your day. The recipes here are divided into Breakfast and Supper, but there's no definitive reason to eat them at those times, other than that they mark a traditional start and end to a day. Many of these recipes work well as anytime meals, to suit the pattern that you have developed. You may wish to skip breakfast, or dodge dinner. That is entirely up to you. The Fast Diet has been called the ultimate flexible diet with good reason.

It is, however, important to aim for as long a Fasting Window between bouts of eating as possible – this is where many of the health benefits of Intermittent Fasting lie, as readers of our first book will already know. On a Fast Day, Michael and I both have breakfast at 7am and supper at 7pm, giving us an ideal 12-hour window. You may opt for something different. We are not dispensing rules, simply suggestions.

It's worth revisiting these words from *The Fast Diet* book: 'Your aim is to carve out a food-free breathing space for your body. Going to 510 calories (or 615 for a man) won't hurt – it won't obliterate a fast. Indeed, the idea of slashing calories to a quarter of your daily intake on a Fast Day is simply one that has been clinically proven to have systemic effects on the metabolism.

While there's no particular "magic" to 500 or 600 calories, do try to stick to these numbers; you need clear parameters to make the strategy effective in the medium term.'

But the crucial thing is to find a way that works for you. Which means you may need to cope with feeling a little…

Hungry?

As many successful fasters now know, hunger is not the beast we imagine it to be; generally, it is manageable, usually fairly modest, and the pangs soon pass. Of course, the whole idea of the Fast Diet is to give your body an occasional break from eating, periods of 'downtime' when it is not having to process food. Some people will find, after trying it for a few weeks, that they can comfortably go up to 12 hours without food. For others this will prove too challenging. The most important thing, remember, is finding a system that you can stick to.

That is why this book does suggest suitable snacks for Fast Day (see page 211). If you must snack, do it with awareness and frugality, avoid quick-release carbs and always keep an eye on the GI. Remember, too, that any snacking will eat into your allotted calories – you will be consuming the same number of calories, but they'll be spread out over the course of the day. Does this undermine the benefits of Intermittent Fasting? We just don't know; the studies have not been done. The important thing, in our view, is not to be put off or to give up at the first hurdle because you find the experience of fasting too difficult. If snacking helps you to start with, that's fine.

Of course, if you eat the right things on a Fast Day, it's possible that you'll escape hunger entirely. Time, then, to introduce the recipes, and how the book works.

THE NUTS AND BOLTS OF THE BOOK

Some of these recipes are gloriously simple; others are more complex. Some are well-known favourites adapted for the Fast Diet, while others introduce new flavour combinations. Some will get you walking, foraging or gardening. Others will send you to the store cupboard for a handful of tins.

- The book is divided into Simple Recipes and Leisurely Recipes, allowing you to spend as much or as little time as you please preparing your Fast Day food

- Each recipe has a clear calorie count per portion, with calorie contents increasing as you go through each chapter. The idea is that you can choose a Breakfast and a Supper in whatever combination you please to arrive at your 500 or 600 'calorie budget' for the day. For good combinations, refer to examples in the Meal Planner on page 212

- Some recipes will serve two or more – simply because the cooking method works better that way (it's difficult to make a sauce work for one) – but the calorie count is always for a single portion. Feel free to bump up the leafy veg in most of the recipes; it won't make much difference to overall calorie intake, but will add bulk and welcome nutrients

- Each recipe clearly shows its Nutritional Bonus (or 'NB'), together with a GI or GL score where useful

Finding flavour without fat

We all know that adding a generous slab of butter to almost anything – old boots included – will make it taste fantastic. Our job here is to fill the flavour vacuum with something other than saturated fat. In this race, the humble lemon is in pole position: lemon juice is a remarkable flavour enhancer, capable of lending a sticky goodness to countless slow-cooked savoury dishes. Roasted garlic is similarly delicious.

You'll discover that plenty of the Fast Day recipes in this book depend on the Fantastic Five – lime juice, soy sauce, fresh ginger, garlic and Thai fish sauce – a combination known as *nam jim* which delivers a mighty burst of flavour with the merest suggestion of calories. Herbs and spices should also feature heavily in Fast Day cooking. Cumin seeds, cardamom pods, sweet Spanish paprika, dense green basil, delicate tendrils of dill… they are not garnishes here, but central to proceedings. Chillies, too, are worth their weight in gold. Here, then, are the basic ingredients for a Fast Day larder:

Carbs
As a rule, avoid white carbs on a Fast Day. If you need a bread substitute, have a thin rye crispbread. And for an alternative to pasta or wheat noodles, try shirataki 'Miracle' noodles. Made from a water-soluble, plant-based fibre called glucomannan, they have no fat, sugar, gluten or starch. No flavour either, so call upon *nam jim*.

Grains
Though carbs are necessarily limited on a Fast Day, those you do eat should be wholegrains – they have more fibre, B vits and other nutrients than refined ones, and take longer to digest. Quinoa is a great source of protein, as is bulgur, while the best rice is brown basmati. Jumbo oats outrank the rest: less processed, more bulky.

Pulses
Legumes, such as lentils, chickpeas, split peas and a whole world of beans, are excellent sources

of plant protein and fibre, and rank low on the GI scale. Chuck cans of pinto, borlotti or butter beans (experiment, you can't really go wrong) into your shopping trolley – you'll find plenty of recipes here to turn a tin into a dinner.

Cans

You won't get far around here without a can of chopped tomatoes, so always have one or two to hand (plus a tube of tomato purée to add base-note depth to all manner of savoury dishes). I particularly like tinned cherry toms, which are sweet and tasty. A couple of cans of tuna (in spring water to minimise calories) and a jar of anchovy fillets? Vital.

Fats

Choose smart fats over sat fats, which means butter must take a back seat. Instead, use:

• **Olive oil:** a monounsaturated oil that is more resistant to the damaging effects of heat than polyunsaturated oils such as corn oil. A recent study from the University of Munich found that olive oil keeps you feeling fuller longer.[10] You only need expensive extra-virgin olive oil for salad dressings and drizzling; use standard olive oil for cooking

• **Unrefined flaxseed oil:** flaxseeds are rich in alpha linolenic acid (an omega-3 fat) and are a condensed source of anti-viral, antioxidant lignans. Use cold-pressed flaxseed oil for salad dressings (don't cook with it or you'll annihilate the goodness)

• **Coconut oil:** slower to oxidise and less damaged by heat than other cooking oils; a good source of heart-healthy fatty acids, it shouldn't your raise cholesterol

• **Rapeseed oil:** only 7% saturated fat (butter is 51%), and, unlike olive oil, it doesn't degrade at high heat, so one for the wok

Dairy

Steer clear of heavy dairy on a Fast Day. Some recipes in this book call for half-fat crème fraîche or low-fat natural yoghurt. It's worth noting that certain cheeses are lower calorie than others: feta, for example, is made from sheep's milk and is a good source of protein, calcium and vitamin B12. Low-fat mozzarella is a handy staple too.

Seeds

Sunflower and pumpkin seeds are nutritious additions to morning muesli and salad suppers, bringing good plant fats to your diet.

Nuts

Nuts are satiating, full of fibre, and handy to have around when hunger calls. Though generally calorific, it's worth keeping packets of pine nuts, almonds, pistachios and walnuts (rich in omega-9s) to add to salads and porridge.

Flavourings

Your own tastes will dictate exactly what you keep on this shelf. Mine would include:

Marmite, Oxo and stock cubes

Spices As many as you can usefully own without anyone complaining

Dried chilli flakes, cayenne and smoked paprika

Tabasco and Lea & Perrins Worcestershire Sauce

Garlic Lots of it, plus Crisp Roast Garlic (Ail Roti) from the Garlic Company to sprinkle on pho, fish and summertime salads

Fresh ginger To slice into pretty much anything, from stir-fries to tea

Mustard Of any and all varieties – they do different jobs: spiky yellow English; brown, rounded French; grainy Dijon for mellow bite and texture

Onions, shallots, spring onions The latter give you onion flavour with minimum fuss

Nam pla fish sauce Plus soy sauce (choose a low-sodium version) and mirin

Vinegar White wine, red wine, cider and rice wine: like mustard, vinegars have subtly different roles to play

Easy chilli and garlic For days when you can't be buzzed to chop

Sea salt (or rock salt) and freshly ground black pepper Each has a glorious fragrance and texture

Sweeteners

Avoid refined sugar on a Fast Day. Honey, though natural, will spike your blood sugars. Rather than using lab-developed sugar substitutes, try adding a sprinkling of coconut flakes to breakfast porridge, or use a touch of raw agave nectar: known in Mexico as aguamiel, or 'honey water', agave is a low-GI sweetener produced from a cactus-like plant.

Ten things slim people keep in the fridge

1. Lemons
2. Free-range eggs
3. Half-fat hummus
4. Non-starchy veggies (cauliflower, broccoli, peppers, radishes, cherry toms, celery, cucumber, mushrooms, lettuce, sugar snaps, mangetouts and a bag of young spinach)
5. Feta, cottage cheese and low-fat mozzarella
6. Sprouts – alfalfa, mung, soy and all their friends
7. Pickles – guindillas, jalapeños, cornichons
8. Strawberries
9. Fresh chillies
10. Low-fat natural yoghurt

And what to keep in the freezer...

Root ginger Best grated from frozen
Soffritto Finely diced raw onion, carrot and celery (also known as *mirepoix*), to save time and energy when cooking any number of recipes
Stock In empty (clean) soup and milk cartons
Fresh herbs Frozen in a little water in ice-cube trays
Soup Double the recipe and freeze for another day. Thick soups freeze best; you may want to loosen with more stock once defrosted
Frozen peas, soy beans and broad beans Chuck them into soups, stews and (once blanched) salads
Frozen blueberries A cool little snack (strawberries do not freeze well)

The Fast Day kitchen

The recipes here require little expertise and even less equipment. You may, however, find it handy to have the following stashed somewhere in the kitchen:

Hand blender or 'wand' For blitzing soup
Food processor
Triple-level steamer – bamboo or stainless steel – or a saucepan with a steamer insert
A mezzaluna and a julienne mandolin For shredding veggies
Pestle and mortar For grinding spices
Kitchen paper To absorb excess oil
A grooved griddle pan To allow fat to run off seared meat
Non-stick cookware (including a non-stick wok), tin liners and release non-stick foil To reduce the need for oil
Silicon brush For oiling
Baking parchment For steaming 'en papillote'
A zester, a grater

How to cook Fast: tips, swaps and shortcuts

Oils and fats
- Whichever cooking oil you choose (see page 17 for your best options), a spray will reduce your use. FryLight Olive Oil spray, for example, has less than 1 calorie per spray

- Alternatively, use a silicon brush to apply oil to the pan and dab away excess with kitchen paper

- To stop ingredients sticking, add a little water rather than a slug of oil

Eggs
- Boiling or poaching means you are not adding any Fast Day calories

- A perfectly poached egg has a lovely rounded shape, a soft yet firm white and a deliciously runny yolk. A good trick to achieve poached perfection is to place the whole (very fresh) egg, in its shell, in boiling water for 15 seconds prior to breaking and poaching as normal

- Time is, of course, of the essence when it comes to poaching eggs. You can poach them up to a day in advance: simply slip the cooked eggs into a bowl of cold water, cover and chill. To reheat, drain, cover with boiling water and leave for 2-3 minutes, draining well on kitchen paper

Meat
- Cooking meat and poultry with its skin on will maximise flavour and prevent drying out, but don't eat the skin. Much of the fat lies there

- Roast on a rack over a baking pan to allow excess fat to drip away

- Similarly, a griddle pan channels fat into the grooves and away from your plate – as a bonus, you also get a pretty striped effect

- Whenever possible, cook meat and fish on a barbecue – it's your fat-free summer stand-by

- Swap minced mushrooms or Quorn for beef to decrease your calorie load

- If you do eat beef or lamb, choose 'grass-fed' or 'pasture-raised' meat: it has less fat and more omega-3s than grain-fed meat (and also implies that the animal was humanely raised)

- Extend your meat choices to include lean game. Venison, for example, has a fraction of the fat found in beef

Vegetables
- Scrub vegetables rather than peeling them, as many nutrients are found close to the skin. Eating the skins will add fibre to your diet – see page14.

- Steam vegetables instead of boiling them – or use the microwave; that way their nutrients are more likely to remain intact

- If you do boil vegetables, use as little water as possible and do not overcook them, as this degrades their flavour and nutritional benefit

- When browning and caramelising vegetables, put them in a hot, dry pan and then spray with oil, rather than adding the oil first – this will reduce the amount of oil absorbed during cooking

- To skin tomatoes, perhaps for a soup, cover with boiling water for 30 seconds, then cool a little and peel with a sharp knife or a thumbnail

- To peel garlic, bash the clove with the heel of your hand, or immerse first in warm water for 30 seconds

- To skin roasted peppers, remove blackened and warm from the oven, cover with clingfilm for 10 minutes, then peel

- Don't salt lentils during cooking; it will toughen them up. Season when ready to serve

- As a rule, use fresh herbs rather than dried as they tend to have more flavour and nutrients. Grow them on a windowsill, or keep cut herbs in jugs of water. Alternatively, wrap fresh herbs in just-damp kitchen paper and keep them in the fridge door

Stock
- A good stock is the foundation of countless savoury dishes. You can buy ready-made pouches, but making your own is good for the belly and, it has to be said, good for the soul

- Have stock handy in the freezer; simply heat it up and add frozen veggies or herbs, warm through, and you've got yourself a bowl of Fast Day flavour

- Roasting bones before adding them to the stock pot will boost colour and flavour; a roasted chicken carcass is ideal

- Don't chuck lone bones: freeze them and make a stock when you have a decent pile

- Add bouquet garni for herby depth; make your own by tying a bunch of garden herbs with string, making them easy to fish out when they've done their work

- Adding a teaspoon of vinegar to a stock will aid the extraction of minerals without unduly influencing the flavour

- Simmer slowly – a good stock should not be rushed – though top up with water to ensure the pot doesn't boil dry

- Skim off any fat and froth that rises to the top of the pot. Place kitchen paper on the surface to absorb oils, or chill first to make skimming easier. If keeping a stock for later use, retain the layer of fat on top to protect it in the fridge. Simply skim when you're ready to use

---

Some recipes will get you walking, foraging or gardening. Others will send you to the store cupboard for a handful of tins

---

Soup
- Thicken soup with pulses instead of potatoes. A handful of lentils will do the trick

- Gravitate towards clear vegetable broths. Miso soup and pho are lower in calories than dense chowders, bisques and cream soups

- Veg stock generally has a lower fat content than chicken stock

- If it suits the recipe, leave veggies whole rather than blitzing

- Make soup in generous batches and freeze – smooth, thick soups perform best – and remember that soups, like stews, often taste better the next day

- Add miso, stock cubes or bouillon powder to capitalise on taste

- When making a soup base, don't sweat veg in butter; use water or a spray of oil

- If you're not adding fat, you do need to add flavour – chilli flakes, cumin, star anise, cloves, a squeeze of lemon, handfuls of herbs – these will all make your soup bowl sing

- A pinch of sugar will bring out the flavour in tomato-based soups

- Use a leftover heel of Parmesan to impart a dense savoury richness to your soup stock at negligible calorie cost

And, finally, Really Lazy Fast Day Food

If all this cooking sounds like too much of a commitment on a day when you really don't want to think about food, there are options that are so simple that you barely need to be conscious to get them into your mouth. I would include:

- Raw veggies – carrot batons in a bag will do – plus a mini pot of hummus

- Low GI fruit such as strawberries, cherries, apples and pears (eat the core)

- No-sugar Alpen with skimmed milk

- Weight Watchers baked beans

- A cup of Bovril, a bowl of miso soup or Ainsley Harriott's Szechuan Hot & Sour Cup Soup (62 cals)

- A hardboiled egg

- A grab of salad leaves from a bag, defrosted prawns from the freezer, a good squeeze of lemon, salt, pepper and chilli flakes

- A pile of lightly boiled veg – anything you may find in the fridge – with lots of black pepper and a good grating of Parmesan or pecorino

- A smoked mackerel fillet with a ripe, sliced beef tomato

- Soup from a shop. New Covent Garden Pea and Mint, for example, has 147 calories in half a carton; for Minestrone, the count is 102

- Supermarket low-calorie meal ranges. Look for M&S's Simply Fuller Longer and Count on Us, Asda's Good for You!, Tesco's Eat, Live, Enjoy, Sainsbury's Be Good to Yourself, Morrison's Eat Smart… It's an expensive way to get a Fast Day fix, but the labels are clear and the nutrition should be balanced

- Other shop-bought quickies: if you are nipping out from the office on a Fast Day, there are good options available, as long as you choose wisely:

At Pret A Manger, you might go for Skinny Dips and Yoghurt (89 calories), a Strawberry Pret Pot (127), or something from the No Bread range (the Chicken Provencal, for example, has 234 calories).

At Eat, the soups, say, Chicken Pho (96) or Ginger Beef Noodle (111), would be ideal take-home suppers.

At Boots, stick with the Shapers range and avoid bread. The Moroccan Couscous Salad (230), Chicken Caesar (205) or Goat's Cheese and Red Quinoa (210) work well.

Ready-to-go porridge pots will get you off to work in good shape, even if you have to eat them on the train. Try Grasshopper pots – the Coconut and Date Porridge, for example, has 239 calories.

But, of course, so much better to make your own Fast Day food…

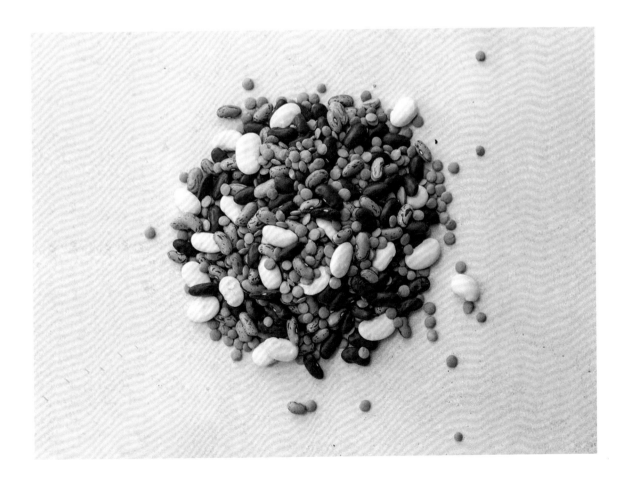

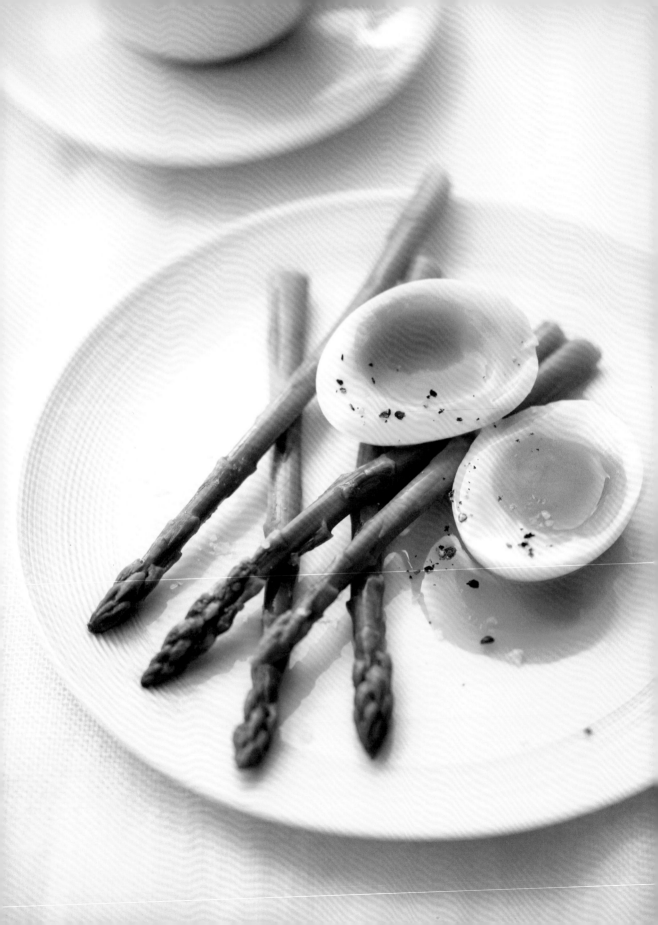

simple breakfasts

SOFT BOILED EGG WITH ASPARAGUS SPEARS

CALORIE COUNT: 90

There's a reason why eggs are such a great start to a Fast Day. They are an incomparable source of good things: healthy fats, protein (all nine essential amino acids), B vits, all manner of minerals. Do, however, buy the best you can – free-range chickens have been shown to produce eggs of higher nutritional quality.[11] Eat them fresh as a daisy, and settle down with asparagus spears in lieu of soldiers on a spring morning.

Take a medium egg, place in a pan of cold water. Bring to the boil and allow to simmer for 3-4 minutes. Take 5 asparagus spears, trim the ends and either add to the boiling water with the egg, or steam for 3-4 minutes.

NB

ASPARAGUS IS A RICH SOURCE OF FOLATE, IMPORTANT FOR THE PRODUCTION OF HEALTHY RED BLOOD CELLS

LEAN EGGS AND HAM

CALORIE COUNT: **118** WITH ONE EGG **193** WITH TWO

Poaching (or boiling) an egg avoids the addition of careless calories. But poaching eggs – like papier mâché, or marriage – is a simple business that can quickly get complicated. The method shown here is the established one, involving a bit of swirling and a dash of vinegar. For a couple of clever alternative methods, and one that allows you to poach eggs in advance, see page 19.

Boil a large pan of lightly salted water and keep at a simmer over a gentle heat. Crack a medium egg into a cup. Swirl the simmering water, add ½ tbsp white wine vinegar to help the egg white coagulate, then gently add the egg. Poach for 2-3 minutes or until set to your liking; remove from the pan with a slotted spoon and set to dry on kitchen paper.

Serve with 2 slices lean ham (approximately 10-15g each), or with steamed asparagus and a scant grating of Parmesan (approximately 1 tsp).

STRAWBERRIES WITH RICOTTA, BLACK PEPPER AND BALSAMIC

CALORIE COUNT: **120**

Strawberries, without sugar, have a low GL and are deliciously low in calories (no wonder many fasters eat a bowl for breakfast). Adding a spoonful of ricotta cheese gives you light-touch dairy protein too. Made from whey, ricotta is relatively low in fat, making it a good alternative to mascarpone in other recipes. If you really want to slash your calories, serve your strawberries with a nubby mound of cottage cheese.

15 strawberries	black pepper
50g full-fat ricotta	balsamic vinegar to taste

Assemble on a plate and tuck in. If you use 50g cottage cheese instead of ricotta, the calorie count drops to 99; with 50g reduced-fat cottage cheese, it's a mere 88.

SMOKED SALMON WITH CAPERS AND RED ONION

CALORIE COUNT: **156**

A classic, of course, best served with a generous squeeze of lemon. Smoked salmon provides plenty of protein, together with important omega-3 fatty acids that can help keep the heart healthy; the capers and red onion here will cut through the smooth oiliness of the fish. For me, the whole event feels like a bit of a treat, which is no bad thing on a Fast Day.

¼ red onion, thinly sliced
100g smoked salmon
1 tsp capers
juice of half a lemon

Place the salmon on a plate and serve with capers, sliced onion and lemon juice.

NB

SALMON PROVIDES SELENIUM, A TRACE MINERAL THAT HELPS TO PROTECT AGAINST FREE-RADICAL DAMAGE

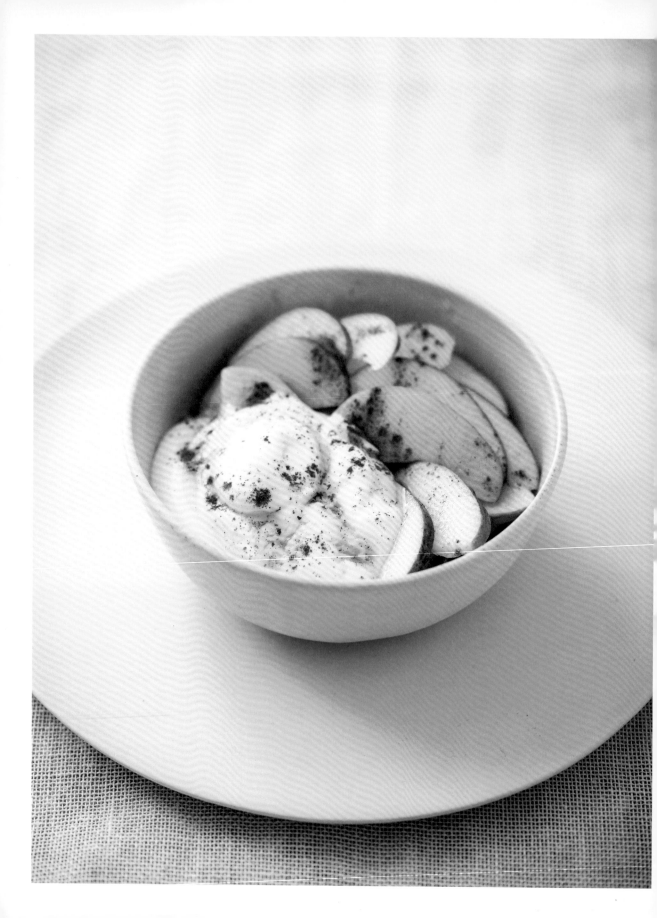

WATERMELON, FRESH FIG AND PARMA HAM

CALORIE COUNT: **185**

Although melons and watermelons tend to be high in sugar, they have a low GL. Watermelon scores a GL of 4, which matches that of apples. Figs are full of fibre (if you eat the skin and the seeds), and they're uncommonly pretty too; a pretty plate is, generally speaking, a healthy one. A couple of slices of Parma ham make this a classic combination, and will deliver a jolt of protein to kick-start the day.

Take a large slice of watermelon (approximately 200g), slice and serve with a quartered fresh fig and 2 slices of Parma ham.

SLICED APPLE WITH CINNAMON DIP

CALORIE COUNT: **223**

Apples are the ultimate convenience food, though they are quite high in calories. Eat the whole thing, skin, pips and core, to get maximum fibre.

1 apple, thinly sliced, with a squeeze of lemon
100g half-fat crème fraîche
½ tsp honey
sprinkling of cinnamon

Assemble in a bowl, and dig in.

NB

PECTIN IN APPLES LIMITS THE AMOUNT OF FAT THAT CELLS CAN ABSORB, AND CAUSES THE STOMACH TO EMPTY MORE SLOWLY, LEAVING YOU FULLER LONGER[12]

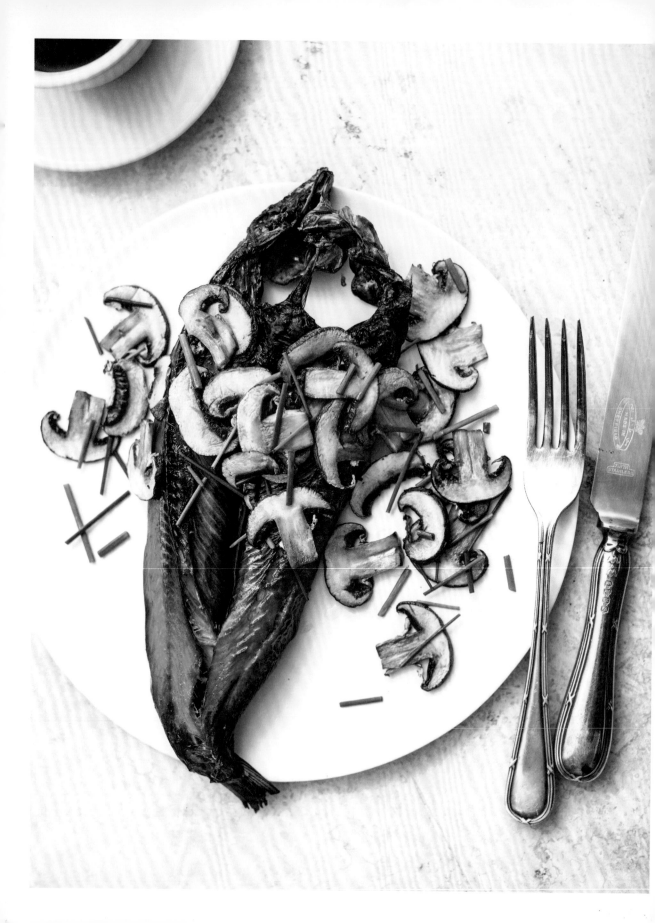

KIPPER AND MUSHROOMS

CALORIE COUNT: **229** OR **234** WITH MUSHROOMS

There is great power in a humble kipper – they are full of good fats and packed with protein. Little wonder they are an increasingly popular breakfast staple. Michael is a big fan.

To cook with no smell, place the fish in an appropriate dish, add a slice of lemon, cover with clingfilm and microwave for 2½ minutes. You could serve with wilted spinach and a poached egg if this is your 'main' Fast Day meal.

100g kipper fillet
5 mushrooms, sliced
snipped chives to serve

Place the kipper fillet under the grill, cooking for 5 minutes on each side. When you turn the fish over, add the sliced mushrooms. Serve with snipped chives.

NB

AS AN OILY FISH, KIPPERS PROVIDE LONG-CHAIN OMEGA-3 FATS

YOGHURT POT WITH PLUM, BLANCHED ALMONDS AND AGAVE NECTAR

CALORIE COUNT: **264**

Yoghurt has long been considered a 'health food' – it is packed with calcium, B vits and friendly bacteria. On a Fast Day, choose wisely: fruit yoghurts can be high in fat and hidden sugars, so go for a low-fat natural version and boost the taste with fresh plums, which are relatively low-calorie and a good source of fibre, which makes them brilliantly satiating.

100g low-fat natural yoghurt
2 plums, stoned and sliced
20g/1 level tbsp blanched almonds
2 tsps raw agave nectar

The ingredients look gorgeous when layered in a glass tumbler. The only other thing you need is a spoon.

NB

ALMONDS ARE A RICH SOURCE OF MAGNESIUM (YOU'LL GET A THIRD OF YOUR RECOMMENDED DAILY AMOUNT FROM JUST 10 OF THEM) – GREAT FOR THE NERVOUS SYSTEM

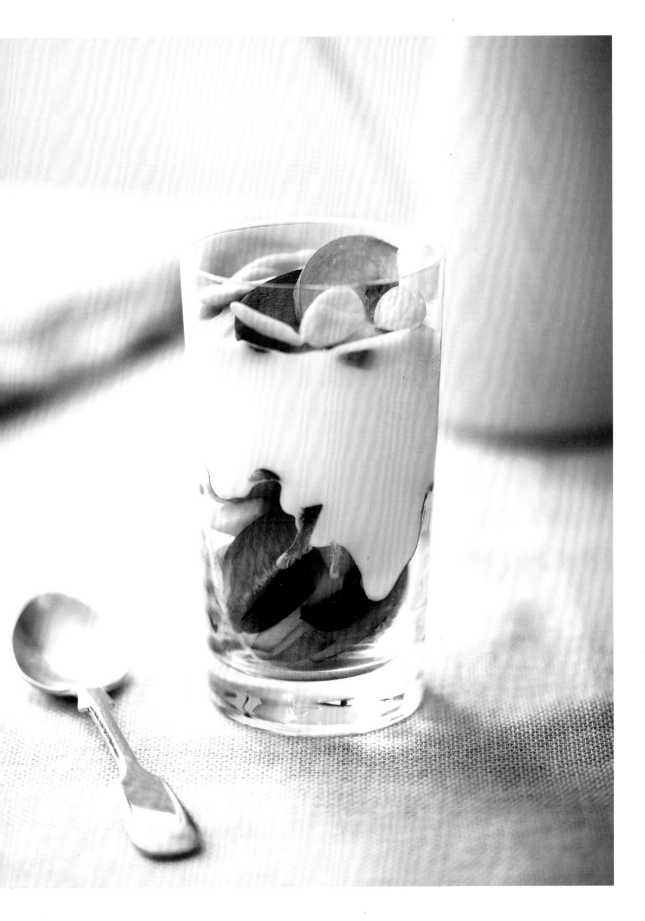

JUMBO PORRIDGE WITH JEWEL FRUITS

CALORIE COUNT: **284**

Add a delicate swirl of pomegranate molasses, along with the seeds and a dusting of cinnamon, to arrive at a wonderful, ruby-studded dish with a flash of inspiration from the Middle East. Use jumbo oats as they promise to keep you fuller longer than the more processed varieties.

300ml skimmed milk
30g jumbo porridge oats
½ tsp ground cinnamon
pinch of sea salt
50g fruit of choice, but stick to the lower
   GI fruits such as berries, cherries and
   pomegranate seeds
1 tsp pomegranate molasses

Heat milk, oats, cinnamon and salt in a pan, stirring well until the porridge is thickened – around 4-5 minutes (you can do this in a microwave, stirring halfway through the 5-minute cooking time). Leave to stand for a minute before adding berries, cherries, pomegranate seeds and molasses.

NB

THE FIBRE IN OATS CAN HELP LOWER BLOOD CHOLESTEROL

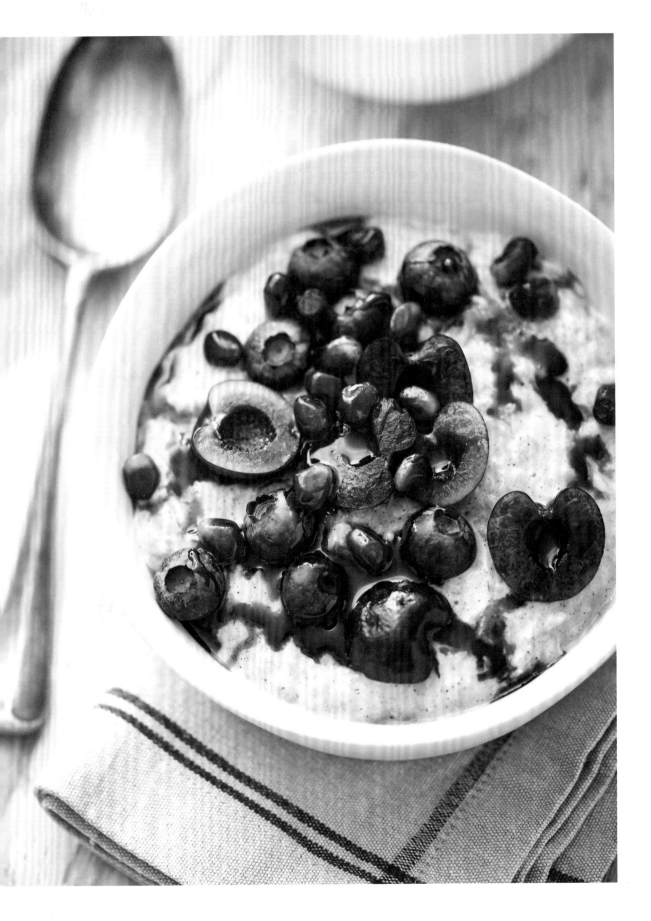

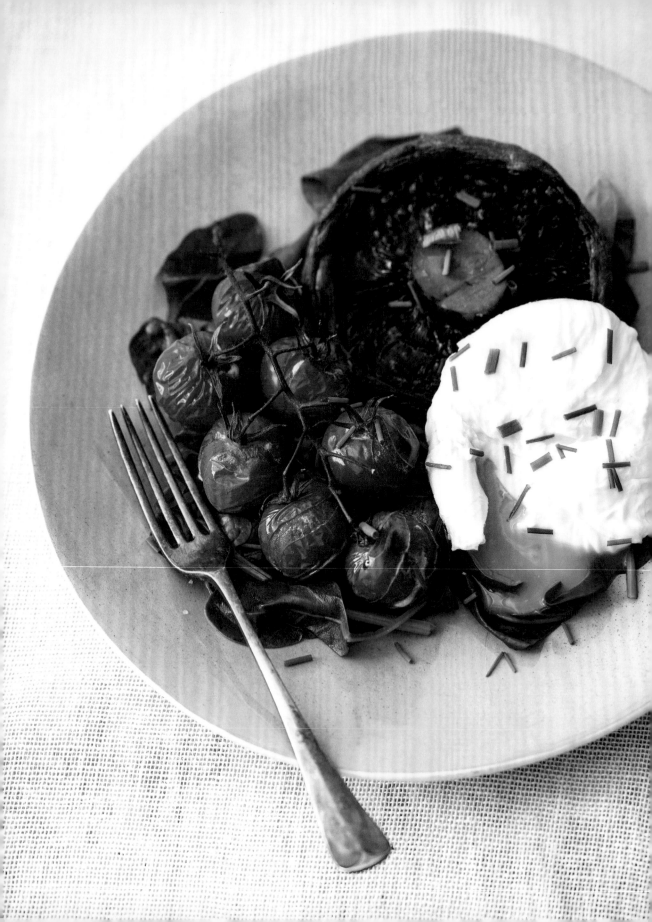

leisurely breakfasts

POACHED EGGS WITH SPINACH, PORTOBELLO MUSHROOM AND VINE TOMATOES

CALORIE COUNT: **124** WITH ONE EGG **199** WITH TWO

Research recently found that people who consume egg protein for breakfast are more likely to feel full during the day than those whose breakfasts contain wheat protein[13], so an omelette makes perfect Fast Day sense. It's the combination of plants and proteins which makes this dish such an ideal choice. That, and the delicious taste – all for obligingly few calories.

1 large Portobello mushroom
1 vine of cherry tomatoes
salt and pepper
oil for spraying
1 or 2 eggs
100g young spinach leaves
pinch of nutmeg
snipped chives

Season the mushroom and tomatoes, spray with a little oil and place under a hot grill for 5 minutes. Poach the eggs for 3-4 minutes (see page 24). Meanwhile, wilt the spinach in a saucepan; drain well and add a pinch of nutmeg. Serve garnished with chives.

NB

SPINACH IS PACKED WITH VITAMINS AND MINERALS, INCLUDING FOLATE AND IRON

SHAKSHOUKA

CALORIE COUNT: **178**

This is a delicious feast of eggs, originally Tunisian, poached in a cumin-infused tomato concasse. Studies have shown that lycopene, a potent antioxidant found in tomatoes, is boosted in cooking, so you are maximising your nutritional benefit with this slow-cooked sauce.[14] The recipe here is for two, as it tends to work better when cooked in a larger pan. Simply halve the quantities and use a small, heavy pan if you're cooking for one.

Serves two

1½ tsps olive oil
½ medium onion, peeled and diced
1 garlic clove, peeled and crushed
1 medium red pepper, chopped
1 400g tin chopped tomatoes
1 tbsp tomato purée
½ tsp paprika
½ tsp chilli powder (mild)
½ tsp ground cumin
pinch of cayenne pepper
salt and pepper
2 eggs
1 tbsp fresh parsley, chopped

Heat a medium-sized sauté pan and warm the olive oil. Add chopped onion and sauté for a few minutes until it begins to soften. Add garlic and chopped pepper, then cook for 5-7 minutes over a medium heat until softened. Stir in the tomatoes and tomato purée, together with the spices, and simmer for a further 5-7 minutes until it starts to reduce. Season, then crack the eggs directly over the tomato mixture. Cover and cook for 10 minutes, or until the egg whites are firm, the yolks still runny and the sauce has slightly reduced. Garnish with flurries of chopped parsley.

NB

THIS BREAKFAST PROVIDES DOUBLE THE RECOMMENDED DAILY AMOUNT OF VITAMIN C

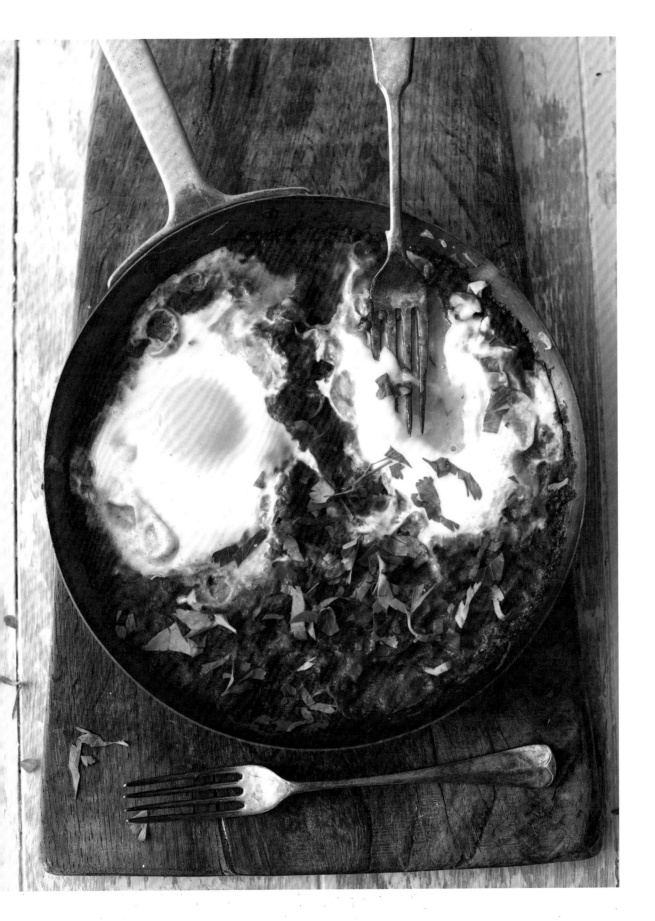

MUSHROOM, PEPPER AND TOMATO CONCASSE WITH THIN RYE CRISPBREAD

CALORIE COUNT: 181

This is another show-stopper, a real 'come-over-to-my-place' breakfast or brunch, which means you can follow your fast without anyone else knowing about it. Make plenty of the concasse – the recipe here makes enough for four servings but you can double or even triple it, and use it another way on another day. It will keep in the fridge for 3-4 days and freezes well.

For the tomato concasse:
2 red peppers
1 tbsp olive oil
2 garlic cloves, peeled and crushed
1 shallot, diced
4 large, ripe tomatoes, diced
2 tbsps fresh basil leaves
1 tsp dried oregano
salt and pepper
2 tbsps water

For the mushroom base and garnish:
1 medium flat field mushroom
1 tsp pine nuts, dry fried
flat-leaf parsley, chopped
2 thin rye crispbreads, such as
    Wasa Delikatess

Start with the concasse. Roast red peppers in a hot oven (200°C/400°F) until browned. Chop, deseed and set aside. Heat olive oil in a small saucepan, add garlic and shallot; sweat until softened. Add tomatoes, herbs, roasted pepper, water and seasoning and cook gently for 8-10 minutes until reduced. Allow to cool slightly, then blend in a processor or with a hand blender until coarsely combined.

Oven-bake mushroom on a baking tray for 3-5 minutes. Remove the tray and spoon concasse into the central well of the mushroom. Bake for a further 5 minutes. Sprinkle with toasted pine nuts and serve with chopped parsley and crispbread dippers.

NB

MUSHROOMS ARE A GOOD SOURCE OF B VITAMINS, PLUS VITAL MINERALS SELENIUM, COPPER AND POTASSIUM

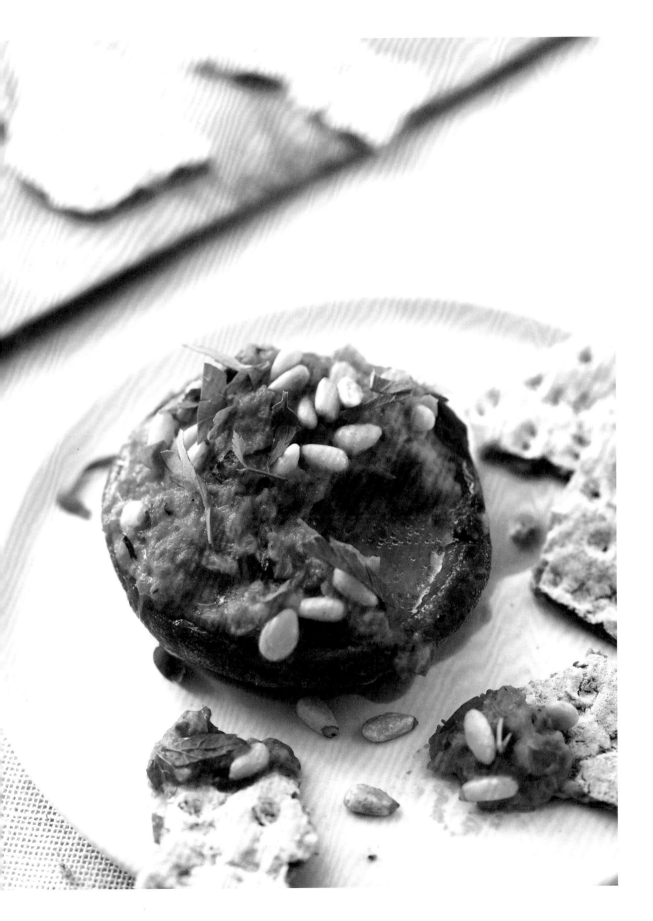

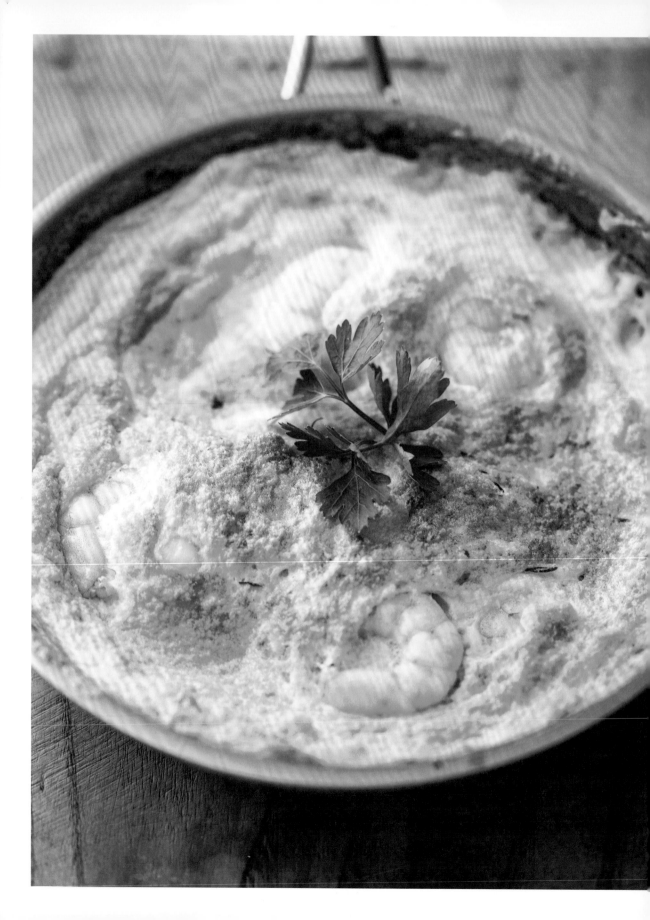

FLUFFED PRAWN OMELETTE

CALORIE COUNT: 207

The fluffing here won't do anything to reduce the calorie count – the world doesn't work like that – but it does look great and it certainly assists, together with the bulk of the courgette and protein from the prawns, in making a substantial breakfast. This is a good one to serve to non-fasting friends on your Fast Day. Let them have theirs with hot buttered toast, knowing that you can have yours tomorrow.

30g prawns, cooked and peeled
½ courgette, grated
2 medium eggs, separated
dash of Tabasco
salt and pepper
oil for spraying
parsley to serve

Dry prawns on kitchen paper and squeeze grated courgette to remove excess moisture. Mix together. Whisk egg whites till stiff peaks form. Beat the egg yolks with Tabasco, salt and pepper. With a metal spoon gently fold egg yolk into whisked whites. Heat pan and spray with a little oil. Fry prawn mixture for a minute or two, then add egg mixture and cook until the omelette is set. Finish under the grill if you prefer a firmer texture. Serve with torn parsley.

NB

EGG YOLKS ARE ONE OF THE FEW NATURAL SOURCES OF VITAMIN D IN THE DIET, NECESSARY FOR CALCIUM ABSORPTION AND TO KEEP BONES HEALTHY

FAST DAY MUESLI WITH CHERRY YOGHURT

CALORIE COUNT: **223**

Shop-bought mueslis not only tend to contain sugary dried fruit, they generally include something you don't like very much and have to pick out before you get a dream mouthful. So make your own low-GI muesli with plenty of seeds and nuts. Stick with it: once you've trained your taste buds to enjoy this infinitely superior Fast Day version, the sugared varieties start to taste way too sweet.

For the muesli:
100g whole oat flakes
30g oat bran
2 tbsps each sunflower seeds, pumpkin seeds,
    linseed and poppy seeds
2 tbsps each almonds and hazelnuts
2 tbsps coconut flakes (for sweetness)
50g ground almonds

For the base and topping:
100g low-fat natural yoghurt
10 ripe cherries, stoned, or
10 ripe strawberries

Mix dry ingredients and keep in an airtight container (you can, of course, multiply the quantities). Take low-fat yoghurt and add a handful of the muesli mix (30g), then top with fruit.

NB

COCONUT IS RICH IN POTASSIUM WHICH CAN HELP KEEP BLOOD PRESSURE HEALTHY

THE HIGH-ENERGY BREAKFAST

CALORIE COUNT: **246**

Cameron Diaz apparently eats her supper at breakfast time, which, she says, keeps her going all day: 'I started doing it when I'd go surfing because I could go out for four hours and not get hungry.' So, if you're a big breakfast person, try an upside-down day – if you can face frying garlic in the morning.

Serves two

1½ tsps olive oil
2 skinless chicken breasts, cut into 2cm cubes
salt and pepper
100g broccoli, thinly sliced
100g cooked brown rice (cook the rice in
   stock for better flavour)
2 garlic cloves, peeled and chopped
1 tbsp grated lemon zest
1 whole egg plus 1 egg white, scrambled
2 tbsps fresh lemon juice
handful fresh parsley, chopped

Heat a large frying pan and add olive oil. Add the chicken and season. Cook for 3 minutes, stirring occasionally. Add broccoli and continue cooking for a further 5 minutes or until chicken begins to brown. Add cooked rice, garlic and lemon zest; cook for a further 3 minutes. Scramble eggs in a separate pan, and add to the mixture. Heat for a further 2 minutes until chicken is cooked through. Remove from heat and add lemon juice and plenty of parsley.

NB

THE CALCIUM IN BROCCOLI IS MORE READILY ABSORBED THAN THAT IN OTHER GREEN VEGGIES

JAPANESE BREAKFAST SPECIAL

CALORIE COUNT FOR WHOLE BREAKFAST PER PERSON: 261

This is a Fast Day take on a traditional Japanese breakfast, boycotting the rice, but sticking to the basic components of soup, rolled omelette and fish. It's quite hands-on, so one for a lazy morning. Serve with green tea.

Serves two

Miso soup

CALORIE COUNT: 78

According to legend, miso was a gift from the gods to ensure humanity's health, longevity and happiness. I have no reason to argue.

300ml dashi soup stock (see page 174)
2 tbsps miso paste
100g tofu, cut into chunks
1 spring onion, thinly sliced

Mix 1 tbsp dashi stock with miso paste until it dissolves and set aside. Heat the rest of the dashi till boiling, lower to a simmer and add the tofu. Let it cook for 10 minutes. Add miso mixture and stir. Remove from heat before it boils. Add spring onion and serve.

Tamagoyaki (rolled omelette)

CALORIE COUNT: 93

The traditional rolled omelette is slightly sweet. Exclude the sugar to arrive at a Western version (your calorie count will reduce by around 16).

2 eggs
1 tsp sugar
1½ tsps mirin
1½ tsps soy sauce
salt and pepper
3 tbsps dashi soup stock
½ tsp vegetable oil

Beat the eggs with a fork; add sugar, mirin, soy sauce, salt and pepper and dashi. Blend well. Heat a large pan with the oil and pour in the egg mixture. When just set, roll the omelette and cut into bite-sized pieces.

Steamed salmon

CALORIE COUNT: 90

100g fresh salmon

Lightly steam the fish until cooked to your liking.

NB

THIS BREAKFAST IS FULL OF MINERAL MAGIC – AND A SOUP FOR BREAKFAST HAS BEEN PROVEN TO KEEP YOU FULLER LONGER[15]

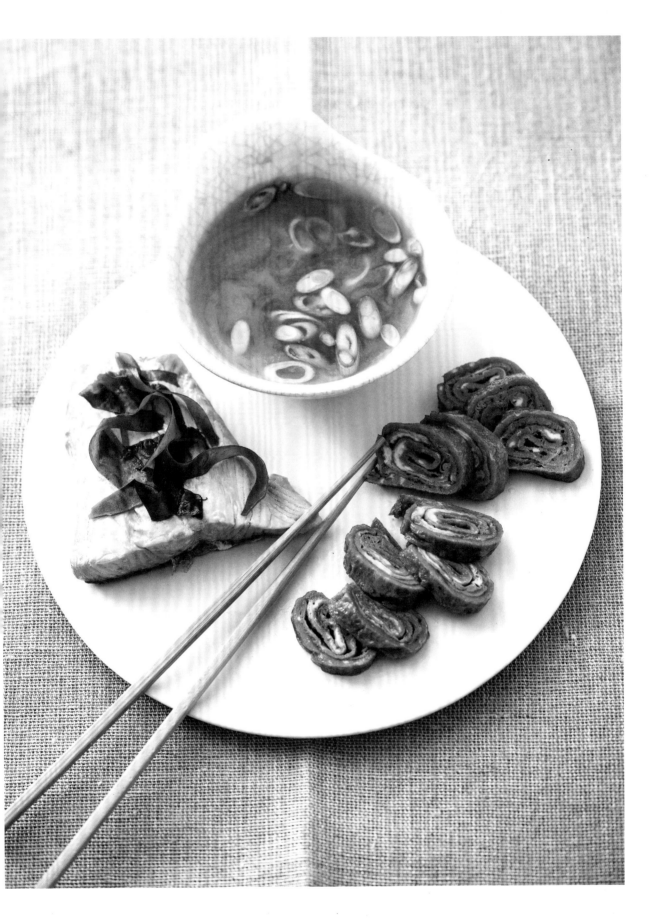

BEAUTY BREAKFAST SHAKE

CALORIE COUNT: **279**

This makes a cool and pleasantly crunchy DIY shake, full of goodies – a bit of a belly boost to start the day. Because you're in charge here, there's no danger of consuming the hidden sugars and preservatives that tend to lurk in commercial products.

1 small tub low-fat yoghurt, mixed with water
   until it's the consistency of a shake
30g jumbo porridge oats
1 tsp sunflower seeds
20g dried apricots, chopped
20g blanched almonds, chopped

Combine ingredients in a bowl or large glass and leave in the fridge overnight, ready for a breakfast boost.

NB

SEEDS AND NUTS ARE A SOURCE OF HEALTHY PLANT FATS, AND A GREAT WAY TO START A FAST DAY

SPICED PEAR PORRIDGE

CALORIE COUNT: **221** OR **299** WITH AGAVE AND NUTS

The spice and fruit here help make up for the lack of added sugar. Oats are full of soluble fibre and release energy slowly to set you up for the day. Add the chopped hazelnuts and raw agave nectar (a low-GI sweetener, now widely available) as a topping if your calorie count allows.

30g jumbo porridge oats
250ml skimmed milk
½ pear, peeled and sliced
½ tsp cinnamon
a grating of nutmeg
1 tbsp chopped hazelnuts
1 tsp raw agave nectar

Place oats, milk, pear, cinnamon and nutmeg in a saucepan and simmer, stirring, until the porridge is thickened to your liking. Serve with nuts, adding a little agave nectar to taste.

NB

OATS ARE SLOW-BURNING AND SPACE-FILLING; THEY ARE HEART-HEALTHY AND ANTIOXIDANT TOO[16]

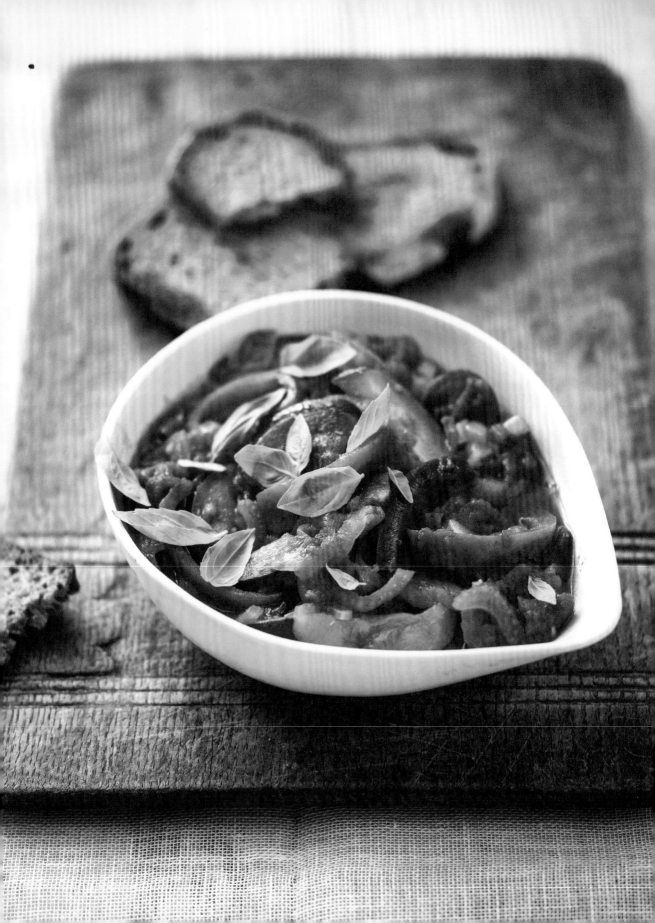

simple suppers

RATATOUILLE WITH RYE BREAD TOAST

CALORIE COUNT: OR WITH RYE TOAST

Most of us know how to make ratatouille, chiefly because it's one of those cheerful dishes that can cope with anything you sling at it. I've slung plenty at this version in order to max out the veg content. Don't dismiss the tiny amount of sugar here – it helps to bring out the flavour in any cooked tomato dish. Make this in double quantity and have it handy in the freezer for a Fast Day fix.

Serves four

2 onions, sliced
1½ tsps olive oil
2 garlic cloves, peeled and crushed
1 celery stalk, finely chopped
2 green peppers, sliced into strips
2 small aubergines, sliced
2 courgettes, cut into chunks

2 400g tins chopped tomatoes
1 tsp oregano
½ tsp chilli flakes
½ tsp caster sugar
salt and pepper
100ml water
handful of fresh basil
4 slices rye bread for toasting

Fry onion in oil until softened and translucent. Add garlic and celery, and cook for a further 2 minutes. Add peppers and cook for 3 minutes. Then add aubergine, courgette, tomatoes, oregano, chilli flakes, sugar, salt and pepper, plus water, and cook for 30 minutes, stirring occasionally, adding more water if necessary to achieve correct consistency. Serve at room temperature, topped with torn basil leaves and thin slices of crisply toasted rye bread.

NB

A PORTION OF RATATOUILLE WILL PROVIDE THREE OF YOUR FIVE A DAY

BEEF CARPACCIO WITH LEMON-DRESSED HERBS

CALORIE COUNT: **144**

If you are feeling adventurous, you could try this (and typically at less calorie cost) with venison fillet. Whatever you choose, use only the freshest, finest, leanest meat. You're not eating much of it, so make it matter.

100g beef carpaccio – raw fillet, sliced paper-thin
squeeze of lemon juice
80g baby herb leaves
salt and pepper
drizzle of olive oil

Lay delicate slices of beef on a plate. Dress with lemon, leaves, flakes of salt and a generous grind of black pepper. A drizzle of good olive oil would make things perfect; add 33 calories per teaspoon if you do.

NB

LEAN BEEF IS A GOOD SOURCE OF EASILY ABSORBED IRON, VITAL FOR HEALTHY BLOOD

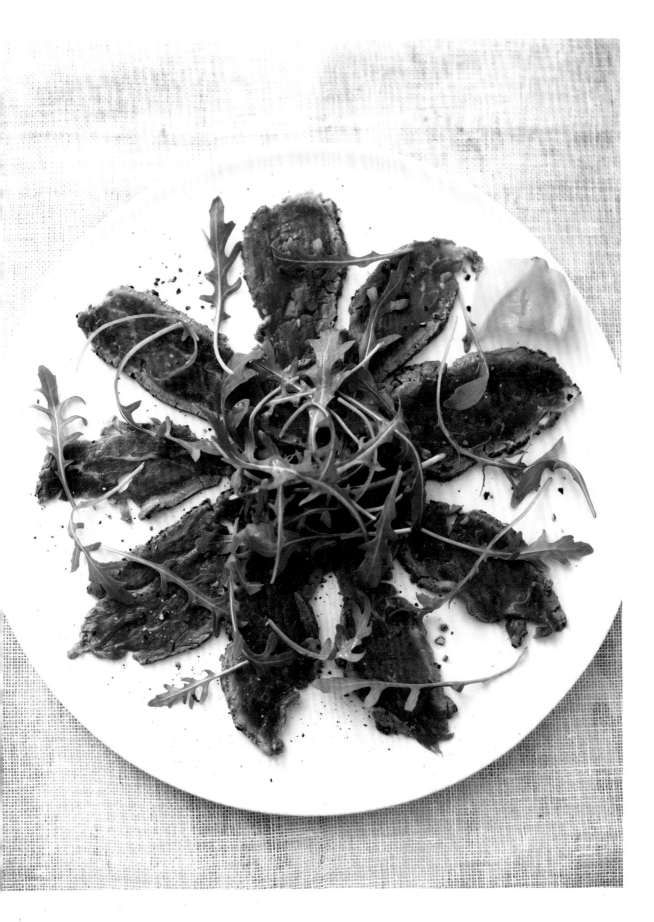

STAND-BY VEGGIE CHILLI

CALORIE COUNT: **149** OR **199** WITH TACO SHELL

A standard way to ferry vegetables into your mouth in a vehicle of fabulous full-on flavour. Don't be too prescriptive here – this is not a bean-counting exercise. And have the taco shell; a bit of crunch on a Fast Day can be welcome indeed. This is another freezer-friendly dish.

Serves four

1 onion, diced
1 tsp olive oil
2 cloves garlic, crushed
2 red chillis, deseeded and finely chopped
2 tsps ground cumin
salt and pepper
pinch of sugar
150g mushrooms, chopped
1 400g tin chopped tomatoes
1 400g tin red kidney beans
1 tbsp tomato purée
100g green beans, blanched
handful of coriander, chopped
1 corn taco shell

Fry onion in olive oil for a few minutes till softened, then add garlic, chilli, cumin and seasoning. Add mushrooms, chopped tomatoes, sugar, kidney beans and tomato purée, stir and simmer for 10 minutes. Add green beans and serve, with a scatter of coriander, in a corn taco shell (which has a low GL of 8 and approximately 50 calories). For a 'chilli con Quorn', use Quorn mince instead of, or in addition to, the mushrooms.

NB

LEAVE MUSHROOMS ON A WINDOWSILL TO EXPOSE THEM TO SUNLIGHT; THIS WILL BOOST THEIR VITAMIN D CONTENT

WARM PUY LENTILS WITH TOMATOES AND CRUMBLED FETA

CALORIE COUNT: **153**

This is one of my all-time favourite recipes and standard fare in our house. I generally make it as a side dish at barbecues, but it works equally well as a main dish, particularly on a Fast Day. Lentils have been part of the human diet since Neolithic times, and with good reason: they are high in protein, fibre, vitamin B and other vitals such as iron and folate – and because they release their energy slowly, they help to keep blood sugar levels in check.

Serves four

100g Puy lentils, rinsed
½ tsp red wine vinegar
1 garlic clove, peeled and left whole
1 bay leaf
3 peppercorns
pinch of caster sugar
475ml cold water
1 medium red onion, finely chopped

2 ripe tomatoes, chopped
1 tbsp balsamic vinegar
½ garlic clove, peeled and finely chopped
1 tbsp olive oil
50g feta cheese
salt and pepper
large handful of flat-leaf parsley, chopped

Place lentils in a pan with vinegar, whole garlic, bay leaf, peppercorns and sugar. Cover with the cold water. Bring to the boil and simmer for 20 minutes, or until lentils are tender but retain their shape. Drain, discard garlic, bay and peppercorns, and leave to cool slightly. Mix remaining ingredients and stir through the warm lentils. Season well and serve with plenty of flat-leaf parsley.

NB

THE VITAMIN C FROM THE PARSLEY AND TOMATOES WILL HELP THE ABSORPTION OF THE IRON FROM THE LENTILS

YOUNG YELLOW COURGETTE WITH FETA, LEMON ZEST AND MINT

CALORIE COUNT: **156**

It's the combination of ingredients here that really makes for something special, the kind of thing you might eat on the terrace of a restaurant overlooking the Aegean… Make sure your courgettes are griddled well and properly striped – that's all part of the presentation.

1 tsp olive oil
2 young yellow courgettes, sliced
    lengthways into strips
salt and pepper
handful of young mint leaves
40g feta cheese, crumbled
zest of a lemon
squeeze of lemon juice
rocket leaves to serve

Heat the oil in a ridged pan and griddle seasoned courgette strips, turning once, until they are prettily striped (3-4 minutes). Don't overcrowd the pan. Serve topped with mint, feta, lemon zest and a squeeze of lemon, with a rocket salad on the side.

NB

ALL COURGETTES ARE A GOOD SOURCE OF VITAMIN A, BUT THE YELLOW ONES CONTAIN MORE

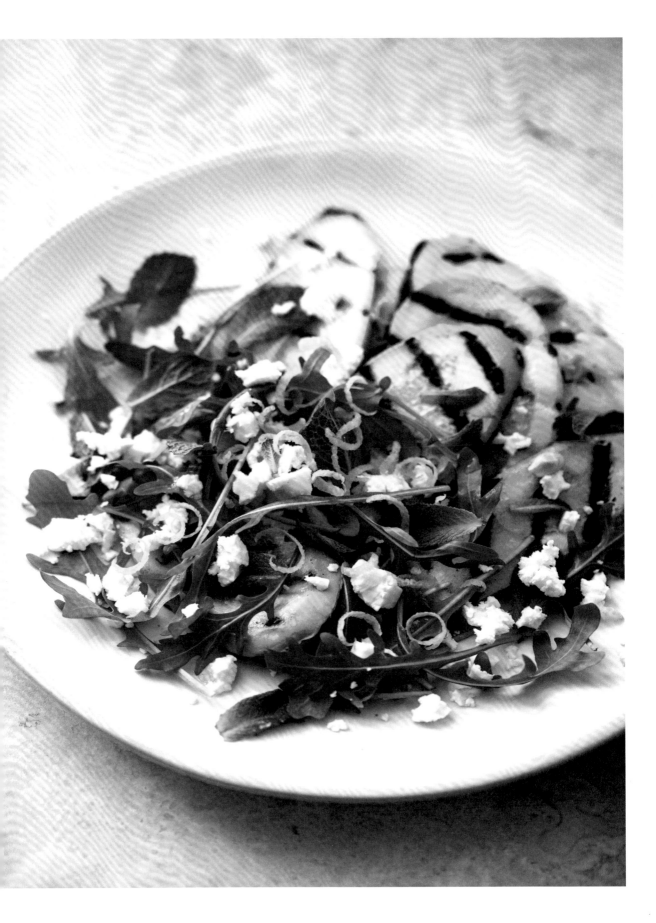

FAST DAY TRICOLORE THREE WAYS

Who can argue with a tricolore? It may well be the most visually gratifying triumvirate of ingredients ever gathered together on a plate. It does matter for taste, however, that your tomatoes are good ones, and that your mozzarella is milky and sensitive to the touch. Half-fat mozzarella will probably have to do for a Fast Day, which is a small price to pay for eating such incomparable deliciousness.

Roasted

CALORIE COUNT: **144**

Take a good-sized stem of cherry tomatoes on the vine and oven-roast for 10 minutes, or until the skins just burst. Serve with basil leaves, a ball of half-fat mozzarella, torn, and drizzle with 1 tbsp black olive tapenade, thinned with 1 tsp olive oil.

With blood orange, rocket and pistachios

CALORIE COUNT: **180**

For a grand and glorious alternative, try tricolore with a ball of half-fat buffalo mozzarella, blood orange segments, wisps of rocket and 10-12 shelled pistachios, all seasoned with sea salt and freshly ground pepper, and dressed with 1 tsp blood orange juice and 1 tsp olive oil.

Classic

CALORIE COUNT: **158**

Take 1 ball half-fat mozzarella, torn, 1 sliced ripe beef tomato and 6 fresh basil leaves. Drizzle with 1 tsp good olive oil and a splash of balsamic vinegar. Season with plenty of freshly ground black pepper and serve. You could add a generous handful of lemon-dressed rocket leaves.

NB

PISTACHIOS CONTAIN MORE POTASSIUM THAN ANY OTHER NUT

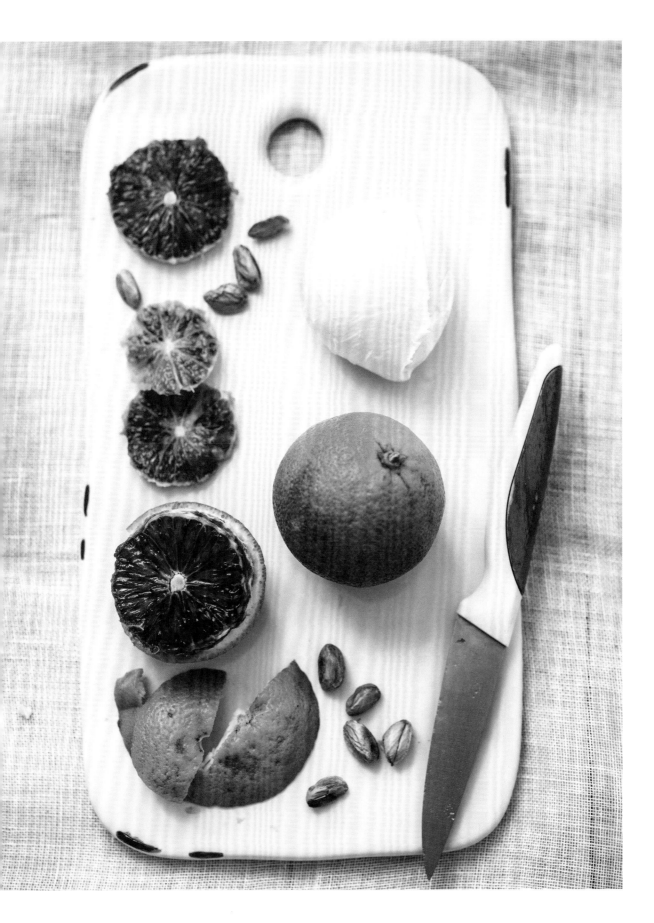

SASHIMI WITH WASABI AND PICKLED GINGER

CALORIE COUNT: **196**

It stands to reason that the pure protein of sashimi is a Fast Day friend, if you pick your fish with care and consideration. Make sure that it is super-fresh – clear-eyed, silver-scaled – and slice it with a very sharp knife. That way, it is a thing of beauty and a joy for about three minutes (it won't last long before your chopsticks get to work).

100g very fresh raw tuna, halibut or salmon, sliced
wasabi, soy sauce and pickled ginger to taste

Place fish slices on a plate. Garnish with wasabi, soy and ginger.

As a great Fast Day alternative, try Italian crudo. Take 100g super-fresh raw fish (line-caught bass, bream, mackerel) and slice it tissue-thin. A sharp Japanese knife, with its slimmer 15-degree angled blade, would be useful here. Serve with a drizzle of olive oil, lemon and fresh herbs rather than the Japanese accompaniments.

NB

SASHIMI IS A GOOD SOURCE OF IODINE, A REGULATOR OF METABOLIC RATE

TORTILLA PIZZETTA THREE WAYS

OK, I'm not about to convince you that this equates to a deep-pan pizza with all the trimmings and extra cheese. But it is a light and pleasing way to entertain your mouth come 7pm on a Fast Day. Make up your own toppings, avoiding the obvious heavyweights like pepperoni. If you want it Hawaiian, be our guest.

For the base use 1 wholemeal tortilla; then top with 2 tbsps passata, salt and pepper and one of the following:

Tapenade, pine nut and marjoram

CALORIE COUNT: 196

1 tbsp tapenade
1 tsp toasted pine nuts
fresh or dried marjoram

Grill for 3-4 minutes.

Feta and black olive

CALORIE COUNT: 218

3 tbsps crumbled feta cheese
6 chopped black olives
oregano and mint leaves

Grill for 3-4 minutes.

Mozzarella and pesto

CALORIE COUNT: 203

½ ball of half-fat mozzarella
2 tsps pesto
torn basil leaves
drizzle of olive oil

Grill for 5 minutes.

NB

PINE NUTS ARE ONE OF THE RICHEST NATURAL SOURCES OF VITAMIN E, WHILE OLIVES CONTAIN HEALTHY MONOUNSATURATED FATS, GOOD FOR THE HEART

SMOKED TROUT AND CELERIAC WITH HORSERADISH CREAM

CALORIE COUNT: 206

The combination of ingredients here makes for a true taste-and-texture sensation – and, with a little pre-planning, it's something you can haul from the fridge on a day when you're pressed for time. The smoked trout delivers a welcome jolt of omega-3 oils, and it's a pretty dish, too. One for a summer's evening.

60g watercress
50g celeriac, finely sliced
100g smoked trout, flaked
1 tbsp low-fat crème fraîche
1 tsp fresh horseradish, finely grated
juice of half a lemon

Place the watercress and celeriac on a plate with the flaked trout on top. Dress with the lemon juice, and a mix of crème fraîche and horseradish.

NB

AIM TO EAT PLENTY OF OILY FISH – THIS SMOKED TROUT WILL COUNT AS ONE OF YOUR WEEKLY PORTIONS

GRAVADLAX WITH QUAIL'S EGGS

CALORIE COUNT: **225**

A classic smoked-fish-and-eggs combo, but with a cute twist. Perhaps serve the eggs with a sprinkle of celery salt. You might like to keep a few hardboiled quail's eggs in the fridge to chaperone you through any hungry moments in the day. Better than Cadbury's Mini Eggs. Almost.

100g shop-bought gravadlax
2 quail's eggs, hardboiled and peeled
sprinkle of celery salt (*optional*)

Place gravadlax on a plate and garnish with halved eggs.

NB

GRAM FOR GRAM, QUAIL'S EGGS HAVE MORE IRON THAN CHICKEN'S EGGS

TWO-EGG OMELETTE FOUR WAYS

An omelette makes a power-packed supper, especially if you combine it with the greens and proteins that should lend your Fast Day a bit of stamina. These two-egg recipes will work equally well as a substantial breakfast. If you want to cut back on calories, a one-egg omelette is still a very fine thing. Or, a one-egg-yolk-two-egg-white omelette will give you a bit more substance without the calories. Simply beat your eggs, and add your chosen ingredients and cook in a pan until set to your liking.

Fresh pea, smoked trout and dill

CALORIE COUNT: 219

2 eggs
25g fresh peas
30g smoked trout
1 tsp fresh dill
salt and pepper

Courgette, goat's cheese and red onion

CALORIE COUNT: 284

2 eggs
1 small courgette, grated and dried well
30g goat's cheese
½ small red onion, finely sliced (approx 30g)
salt and pepper

Wilted spinach, broad beans and pecorino

CALORIE COUNT: 297

100g broad beans, fresh or frozen
2 eggs
60g spinach leaves, washed
flat-leaf parsley, chopped
1 tbsp pecorino cheese, grated
oil for spraying
salt and pepper

Boil broad beans until just tender, drain and run under cold water. Pop them out of their skins. Blanch spinach and squeeze dry on kitchen paper. Beat the eggs, stir in beans, spinach, parsley and cheese. Season. *See picture, right*

Emmental, tomato and rocket

CALORIE COUNT: 300

2 eggs
30g Emmental cheese, grated
1 medium chopped tomato
large handful of rocket leaves

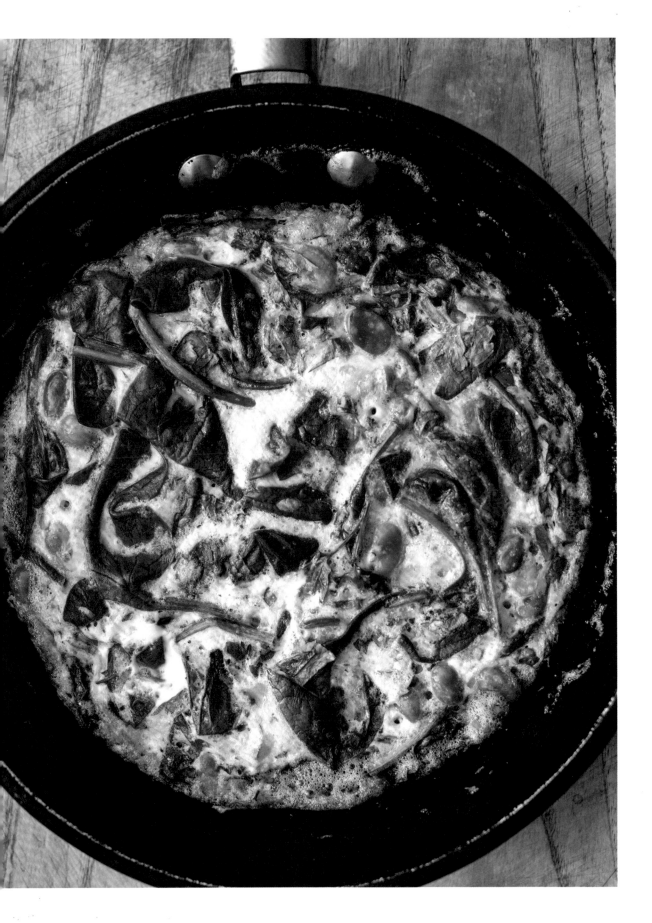

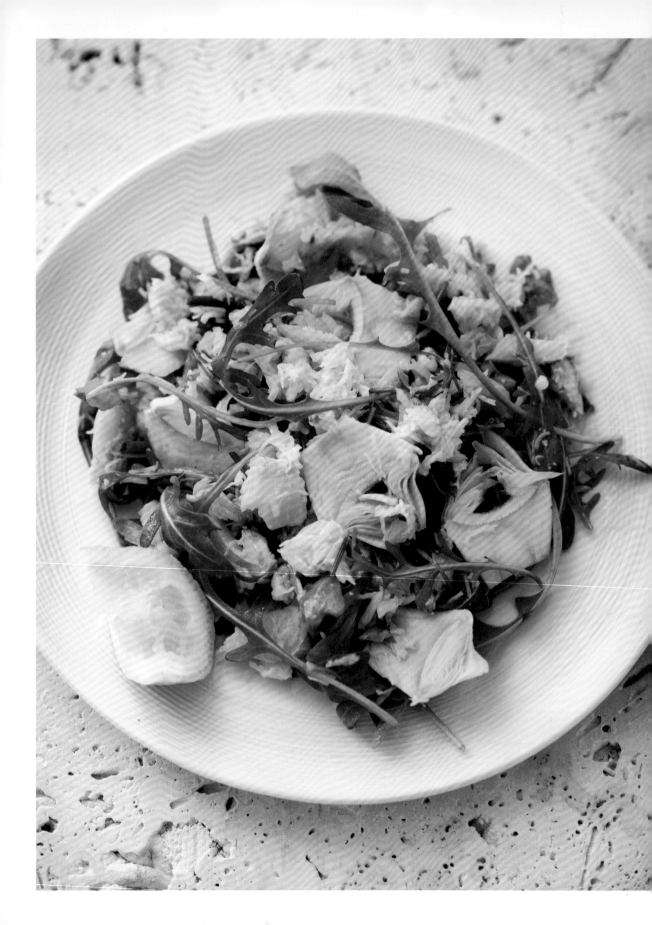

WHITE CRAB AND CHOKES

CALORIE COUNT: **226**

This quick recipe comes from the River Café by way of my sister-in-law Clara, who has adapted the idea to suit her own busy schedule. A pot of handpicked Cornish crab meat is no bad thing to chuck into your shopping trolley: British, tasty, responsible, plentiful and around 87 calories per 100g.

3 baby globe artichokes
juice and zest of a lemon
100g white Cornish crab meat
1 tsp garlic, peeled and crushed
2 tsps snipped chives
salt and pepper
1½ tsps good olive oil
100g rocket leaves

Remove the tough, outer leaves from the artichokes and slice the body of each as thinly as possible. A mandolin works well. Then squeeze on the juice of the lemon to prevent the slices from discolouring. Mix with the crab, garlic, chives, lemon zest, salt and pepper, olive oil and a generous handful of rocket leaves. Serve right away.

NB

GLOBE ARTICHOKES CONTAIN PREBIOTIC SUBSTANCES THAT CAN HELP IMPROVE GUT HEALTH

A SIMPLE BAKED SALMON FILLET FOUR WAYS

CALORIE COUNT: **180** FOR A 100G FILLET

With peppered curly kale

CALORIE COUNT: ADD **33**

Kale is as good a vegetable as ever to grow on earth: packed with vitamins A, C and K, full of beneficial minerals, dark and mysterious and an undisputed star of the winter veg scene. Gwyneth Paltrow apparently swears by it, and I'm not about to argue with the Queen of Green.

Steam 100g kale over boiling water and pepper well before serving.

With a shaved fennel and orange segment salad

CALORIE COUNT: ADD **72**

Fennel and orange have long been firm friends, so bring them together here to give a plain salmon fillet more than a bit on the side: crunch, colour and all-round good vibes.

Take 1 fennel bulb, shaved (a mandolin works well), and combine with 1 orange, peeled and segmented, and its juice. *See picture, right*

With a tangle of steamed samphire

CALORIE COUNT: ADD **49**

Samphire tastes of the sea, looks a picture and is increasingly widely available in fishmongers and supermarkets, making it an ideal buddy for an ordinary salmon fillet.

Lightly steam 100g samphire and introduce it to a little lemon and a lot of pepper. Bliss.

With a warm Puy lentil salad

CALORIE COUNT: ADD **195**

Take 40g Puy lentils and cover with cold water, add ½ chicken or vegetable stock cube. Simmer until tender, drain. Toss together 3 halved cherry tomatoes, finely chopped red onion (30g), ½ tsp crushed garlic, 2 tsps lemon juice, 2 tsps olive oil, chopped coriander, plus sea salt and freshly ground pepper. Stir through the cooling lentils and serve. For a glorified version of this salad, see page 53.

NB

KALE CONTAINS A SUBSTANCE CALLED INDOLE 3 CARBINOL WHICH HAS BEEN SHOWN TO REPAIR DNA IN CELLS AND BLOCK THE GROWTH OF CANCER CELLS[17]

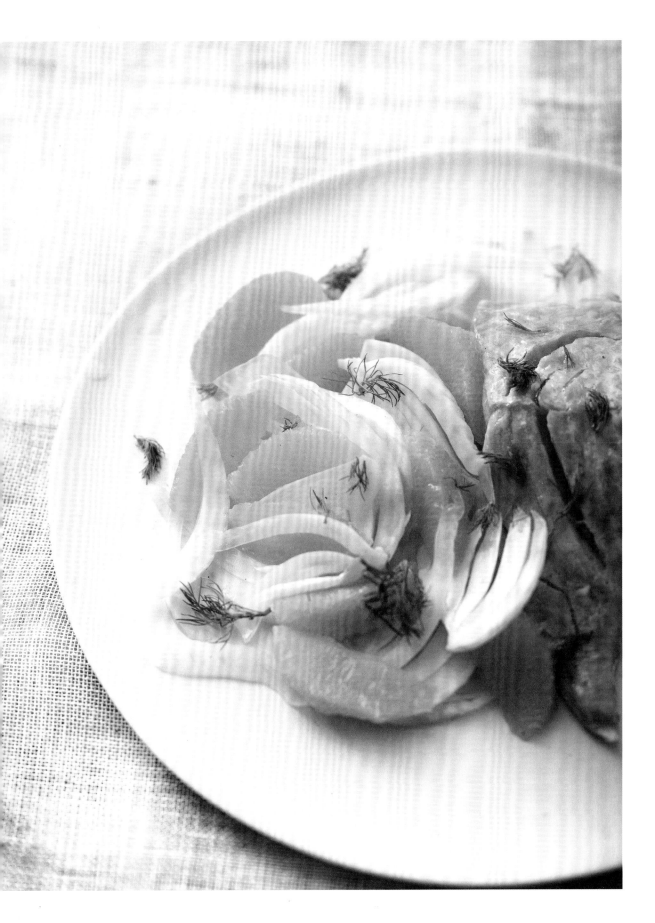

PESTO PRONTO SALMON WITH RIBBON VEG

CALORIE COUNT: **258** OR **327** WITH VEG

A fast, fast Fast Day supper. Choose your salmon well: farmed organic salmon may be your best bet, given that wild Atlantic salmon stocks have been severely depleted, making them not only unsustainable, but expensive and hard to source.

100g salmon fillet
3 tsps pesto
1 courgette, ribboned with a potato peeler
1 red pepper, cut into strips
oil for grilling

Preheat grill to 180°C/350°F. Smear the salmon fillet with pesto (for homemade, see page 205, or use shop-bought). Grill until fish is cooked through, approximately 15-20 minutes.

For the veggies, take the courgette ribbons, red pepper strips and spray with a little oil. Place under grill with the fish for the final 6 minutes of cooking, turning halfway through. Serve the cooked fish on a bed of the soft, charred ribbon veg.

NB

THIS SUPPER CONTAINS 23G OF FAT – BUT MOST OF IT IS THE HEALTHY TYPE (MONOUNSATURATES AND OMEGA-3S)

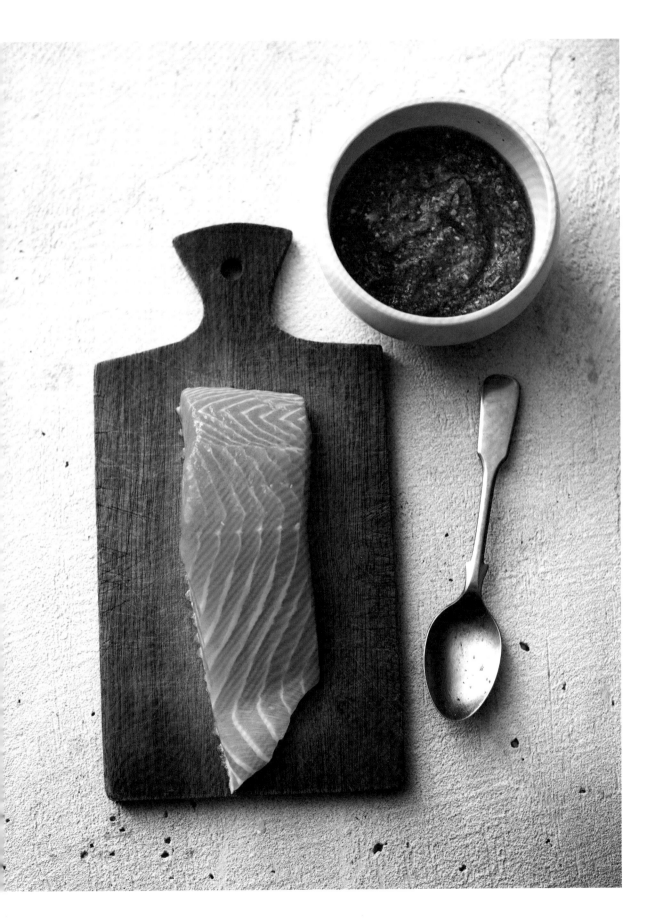

SUPER SIMPLE AUBERGINE CURRY

CALORIE COUNT: **298** OR **355** WITH RICE

This must be the quickest curry this side of a Bradford balti house. There's something pleasing about its humble size and simplicity. But it really performs. It is very good with rice but you could just add leafy vegetables to make it even more Fast Day friendly.

1 small aubergine
1 tbsp curry paste
50ml/4 tbsps vegetable stock
200g low-fat natural yoghurt
handful fresh coriander

Preheat oven to 200°C/400°F. Cut a small aubergine in half lengthways and score the inside quite deeply into cubes, leaving the skin intact, as you would a mango. Spread each cut surface with curry paste. Bake in a small roasting pan for 20-25 minutes, or until the aubergine is soft. Remove from oven and cut into cubes. Return to the pan and add the vegetable stock, yoghurt and coriander. Stir to combine, and cook in the oven until sauce is heated through and a little thicker – about 10 minutes.

Perhaps serve with 1 tbsp cooked brown rice, mixed with 1 tsp cumin seeds, and topped with a scatter of flat-leaf parsley.

NB

AUBERGINES SCORE A LOW 10 ON THE GI SCALE, AND JUST 0.5 ON GL

PIRI PIRI HUMMUS POT, CRUDITÉS, TAHINI, FLAT BREAD DIPPERS, PIMENTOS

CALORIE COUNT: **300**

Raw veg sticks are a no-brainer on a Fast Day. Hummus, meanwhile, scores an astonishing 0 on the GL scale. It's relatively low in calories and high in fibre – a two-tablespoon serving clocks up around 46 calories (depending on type). Go for a light version to further improve the calorie score.

This is not so much a recipe as a loose collection of ingredients that work happily side by side. So play around and mix up your veg: pepper slices, broccoli florets, shredded white or red cabbage, jalapeños, those long, blushing French radishes? All welcome here.

2 tbsps shop-bought Piri Piri hummus
   (or hummus of your choice)
1 carrot, peeled and cut into sticks
¼ cucumber, sliced
1 celery stalk, cut into sticks
1 toasted wholemeal pitta bread,
   cut into fingers
5 pimentos

For the tahini dip:
50ml low-fat natural yoghurt
1 tsp lemon juice
1 tsp tahini paste
1/2 tbsp chopped mint

Combine and serve alongside veggies and dippers on an attractive platter.

NB

HUMMUS IS A GOOD SOURCE OF VITAMIN E – A KEY ANTIOXIDANT

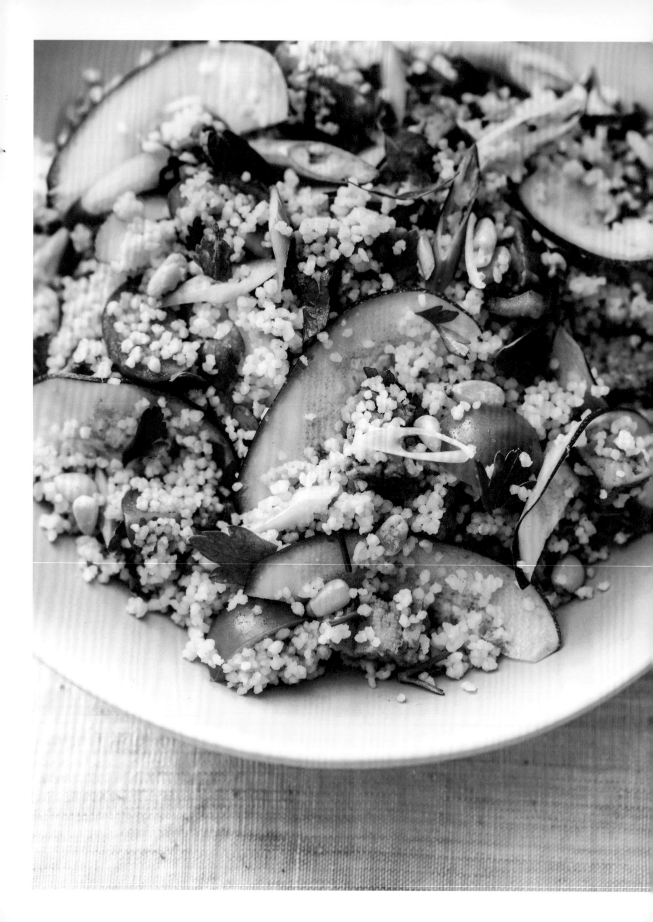

COUSCOUS WITH LEMON AND MIRIN TOFU

CALORIE COUNT: 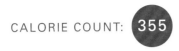 355

This is a complete and filling bowl of food, easy to prepare and attractive to boot. The flavoured couscous here brings an added dimension, though if you make it with bulgar wheat instead of couscous, your GI and GL scores will fall.

50g lemon and coriander couscous
50ml boiling water
1 tsp lemon juice
1 tsp mirin
2 spring onions, diagonally sliced
3 cherry tomatoes, quartered
1 small courgette, finely chopped
20g/2 tbsps pine nuts
1 tsp sesame seeds
salt and pepper
handful of flat-leaf parsley, chopped
75g ready-marinated tofu, cubed

Place couscous in a bowl and add boiling water. Cover and set aside. When ready, fork through and add the remaining ingredients, tofu last.

NB

THIS SUPPER PROVIDES NEARLY HALF A WOMAN'S RECOMMENDED DAILY AMOUNT OF IRON

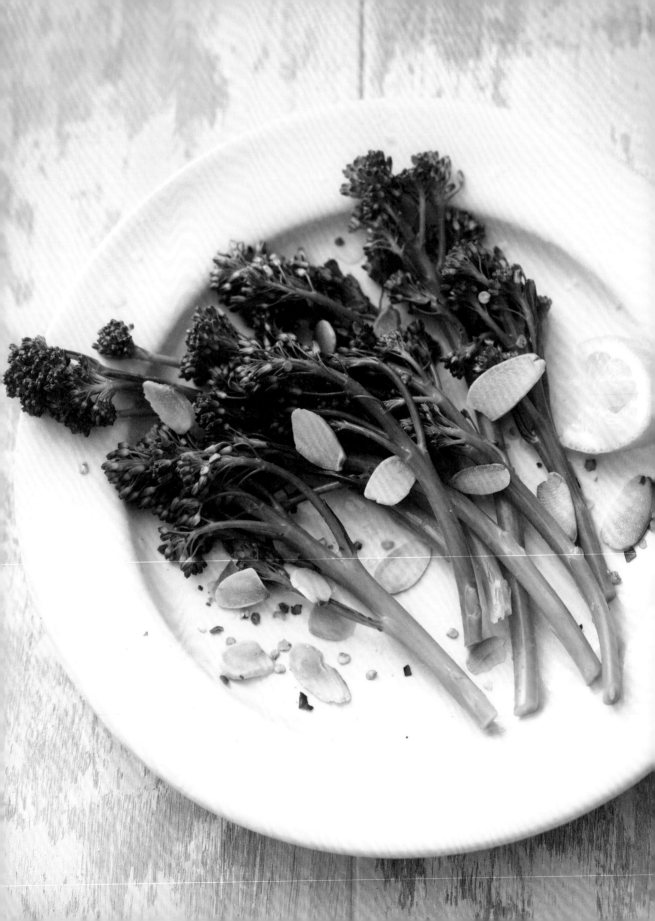

veg

BROCCOLI THREE WAYS

I'm fond of the fact that a whole 'tree' of this wonder veg is known as a 'steam' of broccoli. That's precisely what you should do to it on a Fast Day when, with a little imagination and little effort, you can turn a steam into a superb supper.

Stir-fried with ginger, garlic, soy and nibbed hazelnuts

CALORIE COUNT: 131

Blanch 100g broccoli florets in boiling water, refresh in cold water and drain. Heat a wok with 1 tsp groundnut oil. Lightly fry 1 tsp grated root ginger and 1 tsp crushed garlic, add broccoli florets and chilli flakes, cooking till broccoli is hot but not mushy. Serve topped with 10g/1 tbsp nibbed hazelnuts and rock salt and a splash of soy. This works wonderfully with steamed French beans too.

Steamed tenderstem with chilli, lemon and almonds

CALORIE COUNT: 157

Steam 100g tenderstem broccoli and dress with a squeeze of lemon, a pinch of chilli flakes and 20g/2 tbsp flaked toasted almonds.

Purple sprouting with bagna cauda

CALORIE COUNT: 100

85 FOR 1 TBSP BAGNA CAUDA

Blanch 300g purple sprouting broccoli for 3 minutes, refresh in cold water and drain. Place broccoli in a bowl with ½ tsp chilli flakes, 1½ tsps good olive oil, and 1 tbsp lemon juice. Season with sea salt and freshly ground black pepper and serve drizzled with bagna cauda (see page 84).

For a simple alternative, serve steamed broccoli with a finely chopped anchovy fillet, chopped olives, chilli flakes and a squeeze of lemon.

CALABAZA CON ACELGAS
(Pumpkin with rainbow chard and wild mushrooms)

CALORIE COUNT: **133**

A Mexican tapas dish that ticks all the Fast Day boxes, delivering a great cargo of veg blessed with tons of flavour. Try it with other squashes: butternut and pattypan spring to mind.

Serves two

400g pumpkin
1½ tsps olive oil
salt and pepper
½ tsp oregano
½ tsp ground cumin
½ red onion, diced
1 garlic clove, peeled and crushed
1 tsp fresh chilli, finely chopped
75g wild mushrooms, chopped
100g rainbow chard, leaves and stalks, roughly chopped
20g/1½ tbsps pumpkin seeds, dry-fried
handful of coriander

Heat oven to 180°C/350°F. Cut pumpkin into wedges and place in a roasting tray, drizzled with a little olive oil, salt, pepper, oregano and cumin. Roast for 30 minutes, or until softened. Heat the remaining oil and cook onion, garlic and chilli until tender, then add mushrooms and continue cooking until softened. Add chard and cook for 5-6 minutes. Serve spiced pumpkin wedges with the chard mixture, a scatter of pumpkin seeds and fresh coriander.

NB

PUMPKINS ARE FULL OF VITAMIN A IN THE FORM OF BETA CAROTENE AND OTHER CAROTENOIDS WHICH HELP PREVENT OXIDATIVE DAMAGE TO CELLS IN THE BODY

CHILLI CHARD AND CHICKPEAS WITH WHOLE ROASTED GARLIC

CALORIE COUNT: 145

For some reason, chard gets a hard time in the veggie chart – which is a shame because it is abundant, inexpensive and fantastically healthy. The chickpeas here will give you a punch of protein, while the chilli lends a further kick. And the garlic? Don't miss out on the garlic, which becomes sweet, sticky and succulent in the oven (it loses its after-taste too).

Serves two

2 whole heads garlic
1 tsp olive oil
200g Swiss chard, stalks removed and chopped, leaves
    rolled and sliced into fine ribbons
salt and pepper
1 garlic clove, peeled and chopped

1 spring onion, finely chopped
½ tsp ground cumin
1 red chilli, finely sliced
200g tinned chickpeas, drained and rinsed
1 tsp lemon juice
grating of lemon zest
pinch of saffron
½ tsp paprika

Preheat oven to 180°C/350°F and roast whole heads of garlic until sweet and sticky – about 25 minutes. You can do this a little in advance. Heat oil in a large pan or wok. Stir-fry chard stalks. Season, then add leaves. Cook until wilted and allow to cool on a side plate. Add chopped garlic, spring onion, cumin and chilli to the same pan. Fry for a minute, then add chickpeas, lemon juice and zest, saffron and paprika. Return the chard to the pan and mix well, being sure to scrape in any stickiness at the bottom of the pan. Serve with the sweet, soft roast garlic.

NB

CHARD IS HIGH IN VITAMINS A, C AND K. VITAMIN K IS NEEDED TO HELP BLOOD CLOT

FIELD MUSHROOMS WITH MOZZARELLA, PECORINO AND SPINACH

CALORIE COUNT: 159

Mushrooms are a good low-calorie substitute for beef,[17] so swap them when you can. This recipe works brilliantly as a breakfast too, and makes good use of spinach, that unmatched Fast Day champion.

100g baby spinach leaves, washed and wilted
½ tsp chilli flakes
1 tsp garlic, crushed
1 large or 2 medium field mushrooms, washed and dried
50g low-fat mozzarella, torn
2 tsps pecorino, grated or shaved
fresh thyme leaves
salt and pepper
salad leaves to serve

Preheat grill to 200°C/400°F. Mix spinach, chilli flakes and garlic in a small bowl and fill cap of mushroom. Place mushroom on grill rack and dot with mozzarella. Scatter with pecorino and thyme leaves, season and grill for 7-10 minutes, or until cheese has melted and mushroom is cooked but still firm. Serve with a handful of dressed salad leaves.

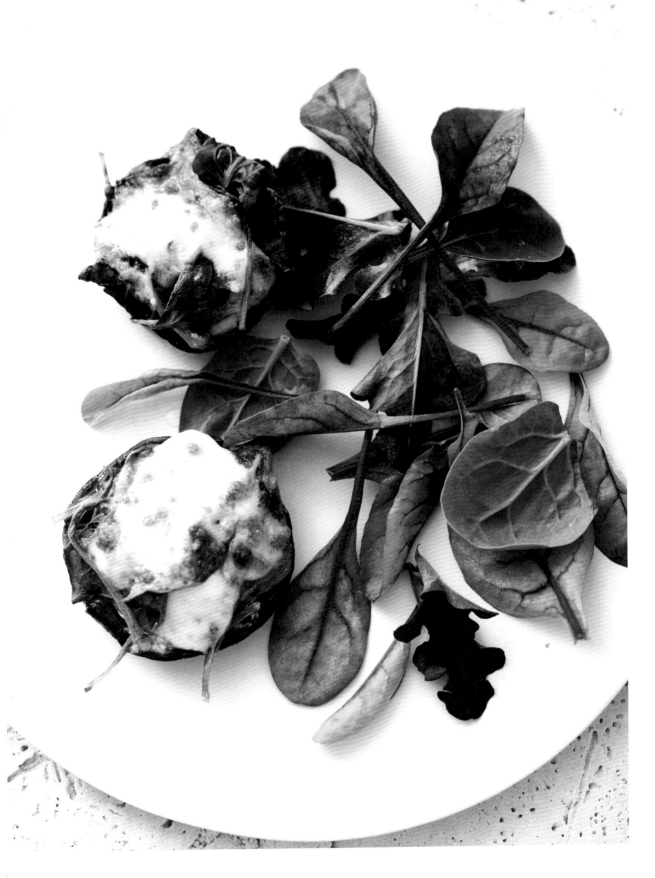

DAHL FOUR WAYS

Small but mighty, lentils are the little emperors of the veg world. They pack protein and soluble fibre all the way, which means they have great satiating properties and an impressive capacity to help stabilise blood sugar. Dahl, then, is dynamite on a Fast Day, or any day.

All dahls can be loosened with vegetable stock to make a soup that is nutritious and heart-warming (a study published in the *Archives of Internal Medicine* confirms that eating high-fibre foods such as lentils helps prevent heart disease).[19]

Red tomato

CALORIE COUNT: 190

Serves two

½ tsp flaxseed oil
1 red onion, thinly sliced
¼ tsp ground turmeric
½ tsp ground cumin
½ tsp black mustard seeds
pinch of chilli flakes
1 garlic clove, peeled and chopped
500g tomatoes, skinned and roughly chopped
75g red lentils
600ml water
salt and pepper
handful of coriander leaves, chopped
chopped tomato and spring onion to serve

Heat oil in a saucepan and brown the onion. Stir in turmeric, cumin, mustard seed and chilli flakes and cook gently for another minute. Add garlic, tomatoes and lentils. Stir in water and simmer for 30 minutes, adding more water if necessary to prevent sticking. Season and serve with coriander, tomato and spring onion.

Green lentil and mint

CALORIE COUNT: 224

Serves four

250g green lentils, rinsed
800ml cold water
1 tsp ground turmeric
1 tbsp sunflower oil
1 tsp cumin seeds
1 white onion, thinly sliced
salt and pepper
mint and parsley to serve

Put lentils in a pan with cold water and bring to the boil. Skim off froth, then stir in the turmeric. Reduce heat and simmer, uncovered, for 15-20 minutes, stirring occasionally until you have a purée. Add a little boiling water if too thick. Heat oil in a small frying pan and fry cumin seeds for a minute, then add onion and sauté for 5 minutes until softened. Add onion mix to cooked lentils. Season and serve topped with plenty of mint and parsley. *See picture, right*

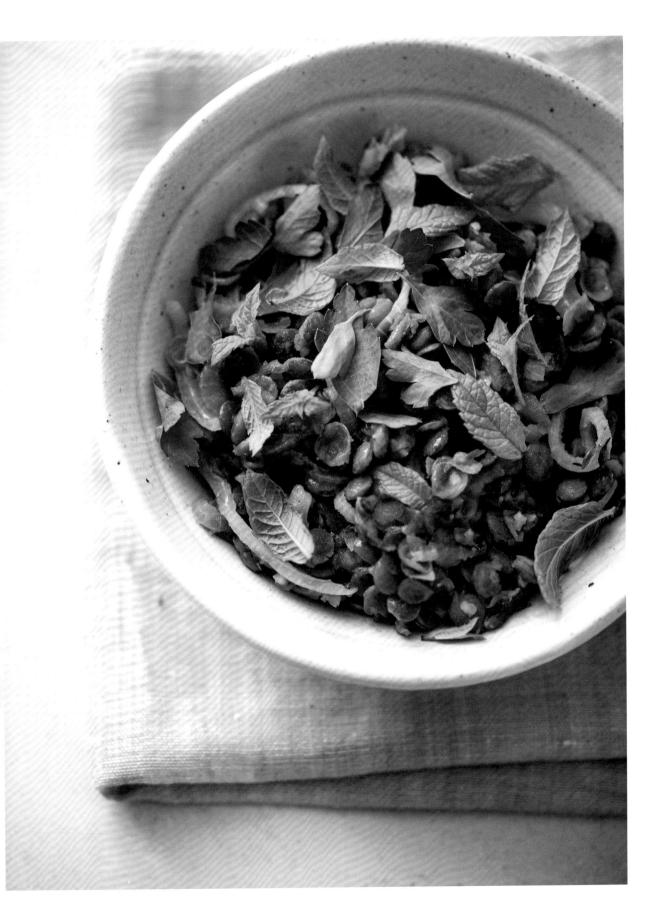

Yellow tarka dahl

CALORIE COUNT: **237**

Serves four

250g chana dahl (yellow dried split peas), rinsed
1 litre water, plus 100ml later
1 tbsp sunflower oil
1 tbsp cumin seeds
1 small onion, diced
3 whole green chillies, slit
2cm root ginger, peeled and julienned
3 garlic cloves, peeled and left whole
3 medium tomatoes
½ tsp ground turmeric
1 tsp garam masala
1 tsp ground coriander
salt and pepper
handful parsley, chopped

Place split peas and water in a pan, stir and bring to the boil. Skim off any froth. Cover and reduce heat. Simmer, stirring regularly, for 35-40 minutes, or until the peas are just tender, adding more water as necessary. Set aside. Heat oil in a pan over a medium heat. Add cumin seeds and fry for 20-30 seconds, then add the onion, chillies and ginger and fry for 4-5 minutes until golden brown. Blitz garlic and tomatoes in a food processor and add purée to the pan, stirring well to combine. Add the ground spices and the 100ml extra water and stir well to combine. Season and simmer for 15 minutes, then skim any oils from the surface. Stir cooked lentils into the sauce, adding more water to loosen if necessary. Heat through and serve with plenty of chopped parsley.

Spinach, pea and lime

CALORIE COUNT: **270**

Serves four

1 tbsp groundnut oil
1 large onion, diced
4 garlic cloves, peeled and crushed
1 red chilli, finely chopped
2 tsps root ginger, grated
½ tsp ground turmeric
½ tsp cayenne pepper
1 tsp paprika
250g red lentils, rinsed
600ml water
2 ripe tomatoes, skinned and roughly chopped
3 tbsps frozen peas
handful of spinach leaves
juice of a lime
salt and pepper

Gently heat oil in a large pan and add onion, garlic, chilli and ginger. Sauté for 5 minutes until softened. Add spices and cook for a further 2 minutes. Add lentils and stir to coat in onion and spice. Add water, stir and bring to the boil. Reduce heat to a simmer and cook for 30 minutes, stirring occasionally so that dahl does not stick, adding more water if it becomes too thick. Add tomatoes, peas, spinach and lime juice. Heat through, then season and serve with rye barley roti (page 86, add 168 cals) or a low-calorie naan bread (add 120 cals).

SPICY EDAMAME

CALORIE COUNT: **191**

These green soy beans are a decent source of plant protein, fibre and a host of vitamins and minerals. Try this recipe as a delicious side dish to spoon alongside lean meat or fish.

Serves two

2 tsps olive oil
2 shallots, finely sliced
1 tsp root ginger, grated
1 tsp garam masala
½ tsp chilli flakes
200g tinned tomatoes
salt and pepper
200g edamame beans, shelled, fresh or frozen

Heat the olive oil and sauté the shallots until softened. Add ginger, garam masala and chilli flakes. Stir, then add the tomatoes. Cook for 5 minutes until sauce has reduced. Season, add edamame and heat through.

NB

EDAMAME BEANS CONTAIN A GOOD BALANCE OF HEALTHY FATS (INCLUDING OMEGA-3S)

BAGNA CAUDA

CALORIE COUNT PER TBSP BAGNA CAUDA: **85**

OR APPROX **205** WITH GRILLED VEG

This centuries-old Piedmontese sauce is cooked slowly, some might say lovingly, to develop its earthy, pungent flavours. Bagna cauda means 'hot bath' – and that's really what your grilled veg will be getting. Bagna cauda is robust (and calorific), but a little goes a long way, as is the case with anything that involves anchovy. Ricotta is good on the side, and a handful of pine nuts would be welcome too, calories permitting.

For the bagna cauda (makes about 350ml):
1 tbsp butter
15 large garlic cloves, peeled and minced
100g flat anchovy fillets, minced,
  oil reserved
100ml olive oil
350ml whole milk
freshly ground pepper

For the vegetables:
aubergine, in thick slices
cauliflower and broccoli florets, blanched
red and yellow peppers, in strips
fennel bulb, quartered
leeks, washed and cut into chunks
radicchio, quartered
endive, halved
portobello mushrooms
courgettes, halved
onions, quartered
asparagus, just blanched

Melt butter in a heavy saucepan over medium heat. Add garlic and sauté, stirring constantly, for 30 seconds. Reduce heat to low and cook, stirring, for about 5 minutes. Add the anchovies and the reserved oil from the can. Sauté, stirring, for 2 minutes. Add the olive oil and cook gently until the anchovy-garlic mixture is golden brown, about 8 minutes. Do not let it burn. Then add the milk. Bring to the boil, reduce heat and simmer, whisking occasionally, for 20 minutes. Season generously with pepper. Whisk vigorously to stabilise the emulsion. Pour the sauce into a heat-proof container.

Meanwhile, roast or grill the vegetables – sprayed with olive oil and seasoned – for 20 minutes, adding the asparagus for the final 10 minutes. Serve each portion with a tablespoon of bagna cauda spooned over and topped with fresh herb leaves. It's meant to look rustic and improvised, so don't be too particular.

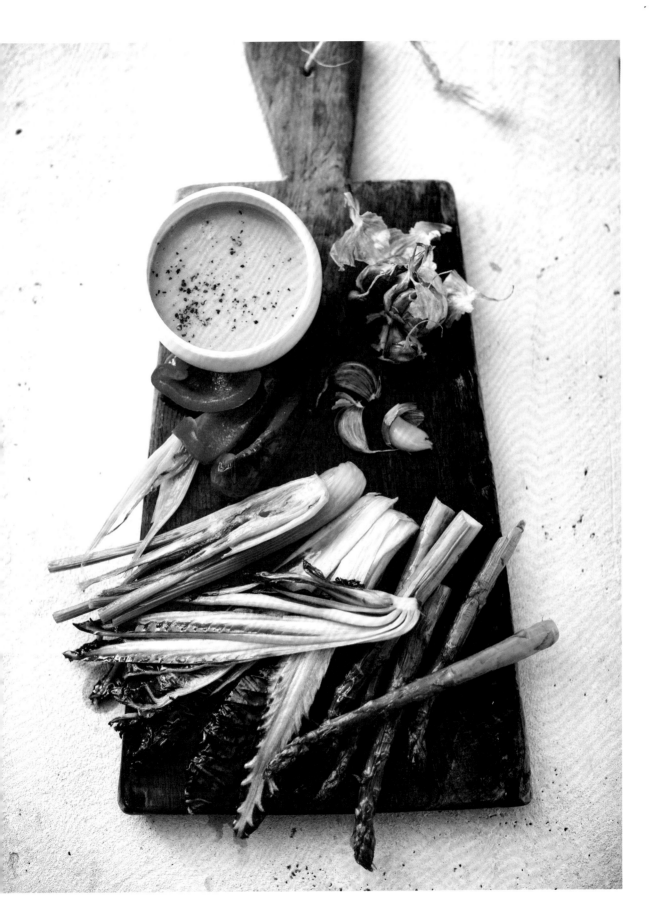

RED LENTIL TIKKA MASALA WITH RYE BARLEY ROTI

CALORIE COUNT: 218

OR 386 WITH ROTI

Utterly delicious and authentically spicy. Really, who needs chicken? You may not need the roti either – though it's a great bonus if you can spare the calories.

Serves four

For the masala paste:
2 tsps garam masala
2 tsps chilli flakes
2 tsps smoked paprika
1 tsp cumin seeds, dry-fried and ground
1 tsp coriander seed, dry-fried and ground
2cm root ginger, peeled and grated
1 tbsp groundnut oil
2 tbsps tomato purée
salt and pepper
handful of fresh coriander

For the curry:
1½ tsps groundnut oil
1 red onion, diced
2 tbsps masala paste
1 garlic clove, crushed
1 400g tin chopped tomatoes
250ml vegetable stock
200g red lentils, rinsed
4 generous handfuls of young spinach leaves, washed (200g)
2 tbsps low-fat natural yoghurt

Pulse the paste ingredients in a processor until well combined and fairly smooth.

Then, for the curry, heat the oil in a large frying pan, add onion and cook until softened, around 3-4 minutes. Add garlic and cook for a further minute. Add masala paste and cook to release flavours, then add tomatoes and vegetable stock and bring to the boil. Add lentils, reduce heat and simmer for 20 minutes. Remove from heat and add spinach leaves, allowing them to wilt in the warmth. If necessary, loosen with a little more hot stock. Serve with a dollop of yoghurt and a warm rye barley roti.

For the rye barley roti:
100g wholewheat flour, 50g barley flour and 50g rye flour (or a total of 200g wholewheat flour)
½ tsp rock salt
pinch chilli powder
1 tsp cumin seeds
½ tsp caraway seeds
1 tsp olive oil
120ml water

Mix ingredients to a smooth dough and rest for 20 minutes. Knead well and divide into 8 balls. Roll each ball into a disc, using a little more wholewheat flour to prevent sticking. Spray a heavy frying pan with a hint of oil and heat rotis on each side until cooked through.

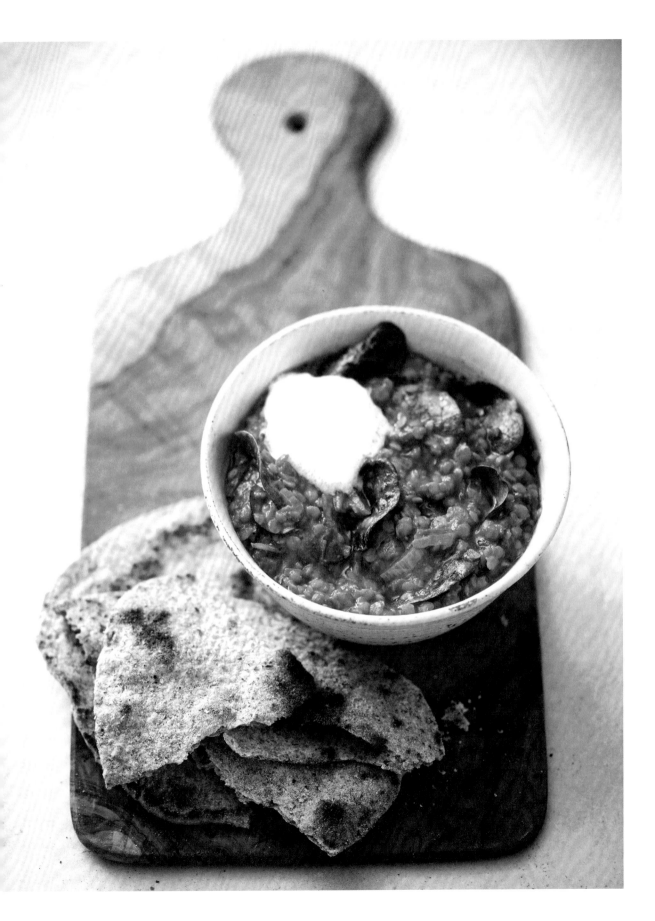

HOT THAI STIR-FRY

CALORIE COUNT: **229**

Here's another opportunity to go wild with greens and consume as many vegetables as you can usefully fit into one sitting. You could eat, say, beansprouts as a panda does bamboo and never really put on any weight (they're around 30 calories per 100g, which is peanuts). The trio of fish sauce, soy and lime juice, plus ginger and chilli, is a total Thai classic and works brilliantly here to deliver super-charged zing.

1 tbsp groundnut oil
60g red cabbage, thinly sliced or mandolined
1 small red onion, thinly sliced
1 carrot, peeled and julienned
60g cauliflower florets
60g broccoli florets
30g mange touts
30g beansprouts
1 garlic clove, peeled and crushed
½ red chilli, finely sliced
1 tsp root ginger, peeled and grated
½ tsp coriander seeds
1 tbsp soy sauce
1 tsp Thai fish sauce
squeeze of lime
unsalted peanuts, chopped, to serve (*optional*)

Heat oil in a wok on high. Add veggies (beansprouts and mangetouts last) and stir-fry for 3 minutes, then add garlic, chilli, ginger and coriander seed and cook for a further few minutes. Add soy sauce, fish sauce and lime for the final minute of cooking and serve, with more fresh beansprouts and chopped peanuts if your calorie count allows (add 73 cals for 10 nuts).

NB

KEEP THE VEGGIES CRUNCHY – IT CAN HELP RETAIN THEIR VITAMIN CONTENT

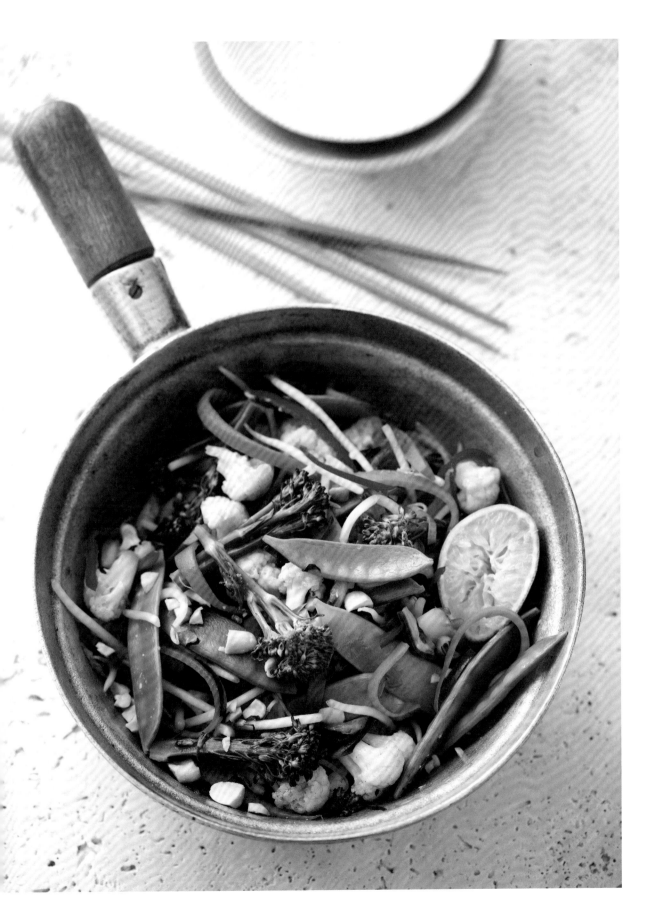

WILD MUSHROOMS WITH SAGE, SOFT POACHED EGG AND PARMESAN

CALORIE COUNT: **236**

For me, wild mushrooms still feel like a mystical treat, with their flavour of the deep woods. Combined with downy sage, a yielding egg and the salt-tang of Parmesan, you have a heavenly plate of food.

1 tsp olive oil
1 small red chilli, finely chopped
½ tsp garlic, crushed
2 sage leaves
100g wild mushrooms, any type, washed and dried
30g dried porcini, softened in a little boiling water for
   30 minutes (save the water), chopped
salt and pepper
1 egg
50g rocket leaves
1 tsp Parmesan shavings and sage leaves to serve

Heat oil in a frying pan and gently fry chilli, garlic and sage for 2 minutes. Add wild mushrooms, porcini and their liquor. Season and set aside. Poach the egg in a large pan of salted boiling water (see page 24) and place on top of warm mushroom mix, combined with rocket leaves. Add Parmesan and torn fresh sage leaves to serve.

NB

WILD MUSHROOMS OFTEN CONTAIN MORE SELENIUM AS THEY GROW IN MINERAL-RICH SOIL

TRIPLE BEAN STEW WITH VANILLA POD AND PANDAN

CALORIE COUNT: **237**

Lots of protein, loads of fibre and plenty of vitamins for very few calories: beans meanz sense on a Fast Day. Jazz them up with unusual flavours: the pandan leaf here, with its smoky notes, is great but optional – though do have a go with the vanilla pod, a surprising and effective pairing that will turn any old bean stew into something altogether more interesting.

Serves four

1 tbsp groundnut oil
2 shallots, finely chopped
1 small leek, washed and finely sliced
1 celery stalk, finely sliced
½ fennel bulb, diced
800g mixed tinned beans –
    perhaps a trio of borlotti, flageolet and haricot
½ pandan leaf, crushed
pinch of chilli flakes
1 bay leaf
200ml vegetable stock
½ vanilla pod
salt and pepper

Heat oil in a large pan and add shallots. Fry for a minute then add the chopped veg. Sauté until softened. Add beans, pandan leaf, chilli flakes and bay, plus vegetable stock. Simmer for 10-15 minutes, allowing stew to reduce a little. Add the seeds scraped from vanilla pod. Season and serve with a steamed dark-green leaf such as kale.

NB

LEGUMES SUCH AS BEANS PROVIDE VITAMIN B6, IMPORTANT FOR CELLULAR FUNCTION AND BRAIN CHEMISTRY

PAN-ROASTED VEG WITH SPICED BALSAMIC GLAZE

CALORIE COUNT: **261** OR **309** WITH GOAT'S CHEESE

This is a premium version of the simple roast veg we endlessly sling in the oven with a 'slug of olive oil'. It amounts to a proper meal in itself, complete with sticky bits, gorgeous balsamic colour and bursts of spiced flavour. Personally, I'd include the goat's cheese and save calories elsewhere; it's too good to miss.

Serves two

½ tsp cumin seeds
½ tsp nigella seeds
½ tsp mustard seeds
1 tbsp olive oil
1 red onion, sliced
3 garlic cloves, peeled and crushed
½ red chilli, finely chopped
1 red, 1 yellow, 1 orange pepper, sliced

1 courgette, thickly sliced
1 small aubergine, thickly sliced
1 small butternut squash, unpeeled,
  deseeded and cubed
fresh marjoram
juice of a lemon
1 tbsp good balsamic vinegar
15g Chèvre Basque and sweet pickled
  guindilla peppers to serve *(optional)*

Preheat oven to 220°C/425°F. In a small frying pan, gently dry-fry seeds, then add oil and onion and cook until softened. Add garlic and chilli and cook for a further 2 minutes. Place vegetables in a roasting pan and stir in the spiced onion mix, marjoram, lemon and balsamic, making sure that everything is well coated. Roast in the oven for 20-30 minutes, until caramelised and sticky. Serve with a peppery green salad, plus a shaving of Chèvre Basque and sweet pickled guindilla peppers.

NB

THESE VIBRANT COLOURS INDICATE PLENTY OF BETA CAROTENE AND OTHER IMPORTANT ANTIOXIDANTS

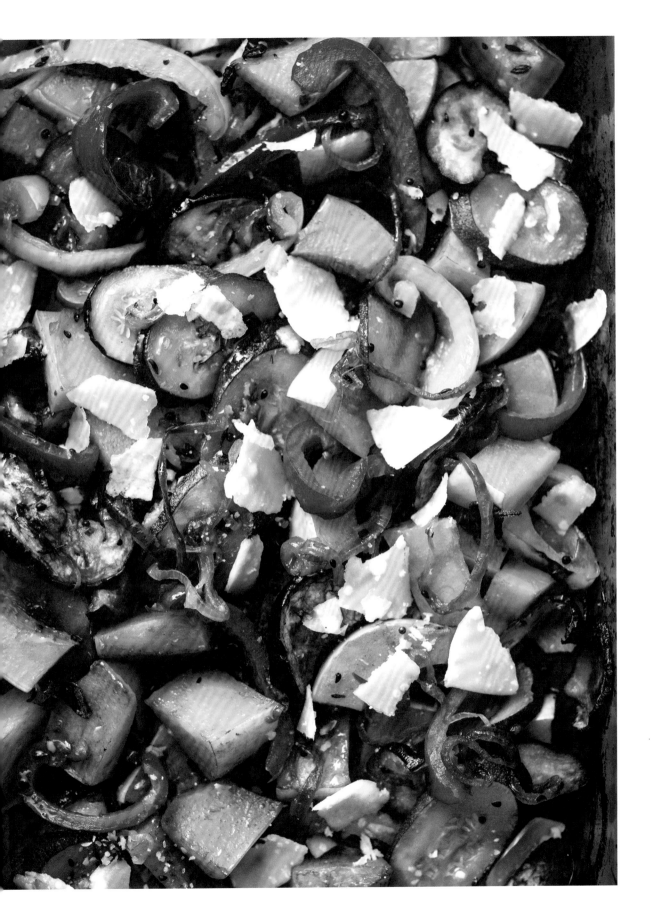

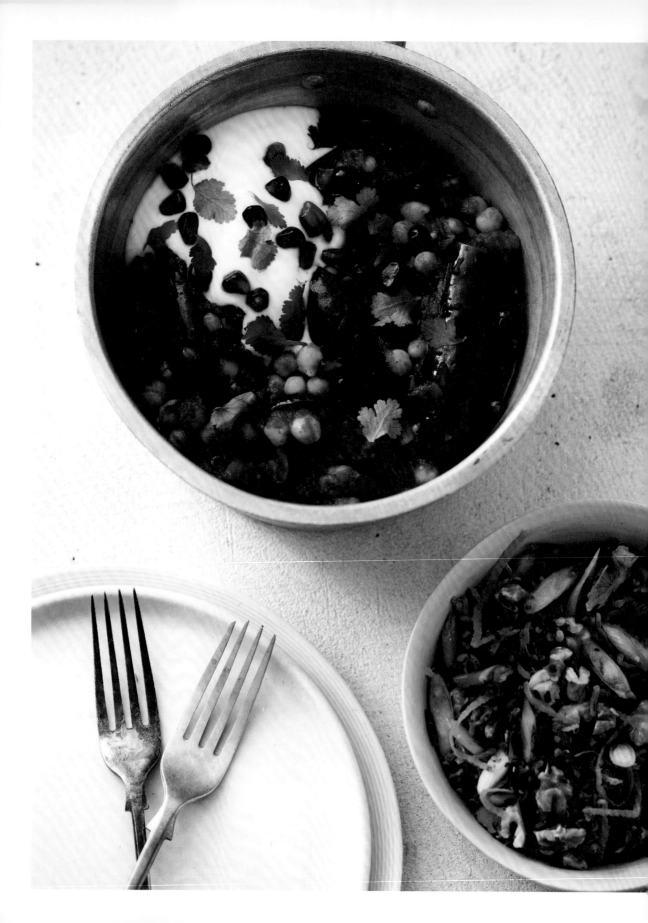

SPICED BABY AUBERGINE WITH POMEGRANATE YOGHURT AND WALNUT RICE

CALORIE COUNT: **298** OR **412** WITH RICE SALAD

No recipe book is complete these days without the obligatory pomegranate seeds scattered over anything that doesn't move – and here they bring a touch of ruby magic to a brilliantly balanced, terrifically appealing dish. The rice, though nice, will whack up the calorie count considerably, so only include it if your budget allows.

Serves two

1 medium onion, chopped
1 tbsp olive oil
1 garlic clove, peeled and crushed
1 tbsp fresh root ginger, grated
1 tbsp harissa paste
2 tsps cumin seeds
2 tsps ground coriander
4 baby aubergines, halved

1 400g tin of chopped tomatoes
1 tbsp tomato purée
squeeze of lemon
½ tsp sugar
salt and pepper
200g tinned chickpeas, drained
fresh coriander leaves, torn
1 tbsp low-fat natural yoghurt
handful of pomegranate seeds

Soften onion in olive oil and add garlic, ginger, harissa, cumin seeds and coriander. Cook for 3 minutes, then add aubergines, chopped tomatoes, tomato purée, lemon, sugar and salt and pepper. Simmer for 30 minutes and add chickpeas, plus 1 tbsp water if sauce is too thick. Heat through and serve with torn coriander and drizzle with low-fat yoghurt, a scatter of pomegranate seeds and a side of nutty wild rice salad.

For the walnut wild rice salad:
50g wild brown rice, cooked until tender,
   drained and cooled
20g walnuts, chopped
1 spring onion, finely chopped

2 tsps grated orange zest
1 tbsp orange juice
½ tsp chilli flakes
coriander leaves, torn
salt and pepper

Combine ingredients, mix and serve, topped with torn coriander.

NB

POMEGRANATES CONTAIN ANTIOXIDANTS WITH THE POTENTIAL TO SCAVENGE FREE RADICALS, WHICH CAUSE DAMAGE TO BODY CELLS

RED VEG GOULASH WITH KOHLRABI AND RADISH SALAD

CALORIE COUNT: **303** OR **325** WITH SALAD

The paprika brings a smoky hum to proceedings here, and again, this recipe gives you a whole world of veg in a bowl. Cut through the dense flavours with a crisp, crunchy salad. And fear not the humble kohlrabi – this knobbly cousin of the cabbage may be commonly used as cattle feed, but it is in fact enormously nutritious, stuffed with minerals and good old-fashioned vitamin C.

Serves four

1 tbsp groundnut oil
2 medium red onions, chopped
1 garlic clove, peeled and halved
2 tsps paprika
1 tsp smoked paprika
2 tsps dried oregano
1 tsp dried basil
2 red peppers, sliced
2 carrots, peeled and thickly sliced

200g butter beans, drained and rinsed
100g tinned kidney beans, drained and rinsed
100g red split lentils, rinsed
4 large ripe tomatoes, skinned and chopped
2 tbsps tomato purée
750ml vegetable stock
150ml red wine
1 whole dried chilli (*optional*)
sea salt and freshly ground pepper

Heat oil in a large heavy saucepan and fry onions till softened. Add garlic and fry for a further minute. Add paprikas, oregano and basil. Stir and add peppers and carrots, cooking for a further 5 minutes. Then add beans, lentils, tomatoes, tomato purée, stock and red wine. Place dried chilli in the broth and simmer for 20 minutes until lentils are cooked through and the dish is thickened.

Serve with a salad of thinly sliced peeled kohlrabi and radish (perhaps red and white mooli), dressed with a vinaigrette made from 2 tsps white wine vinegar, 1 tsp lime juice, 1 tsp groundnut oil, 1 tsp poppy seeds, 1 tsp fennel seeds and a pinch of caster sugar. Garnish with torn flat-leaf parsley.

NB

RADISHES CONTAIN A TYPE OF FIBRE CALLED ARABINOGALACTAN WHICH IS GOOD FOR BOOSTING FRIENDLY BACTERIA IN THE GUT

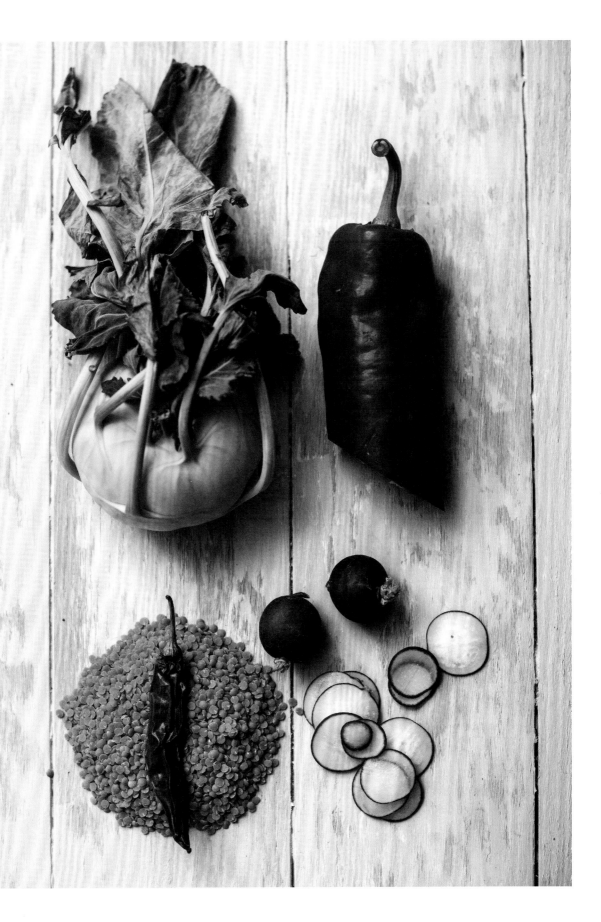

HOT, SWEET AND SOUR TOFU

CALORIE COUNT: **345**

On its own, tofu is nothing special; in fact, it's a bit of a bore. But marinate it and it springs to life, soaking up flavour and bringing fine low-fat protein to your fork. Use firm tofu – the silken variety is best for blending, while the firm should hold its shape in the wok. Firm tofu also tends to contain the most calcium and should be press-dried before cooking or marinating. Searing tofu, just as you would meat, blesses it with a golden exterior and the promise of a wobbling white interior, a fabulous foil to the al dente crunch of the peppers.

1½ tsps groundnut oil
100g firm tofu, cut into cubes or
   slices, press-dried on kitchen paper
1 garlic clove, peeled and crushed
1 spring onion, chopped
2 tsps root ginger, grated
pinch of chilli flakes
50g red or yellow pepper, thinly sliced
50g chestnut mushrooms, sliced
50g broccoli, blanched and refreshed in cold water
50g beansprouts
1 tbsp soy sauce
1 tsp raw agave syrup
squeeze of lemon

Heat oil in a wok. Fry tofu cubes till golden and gently set aside on kitchen paper. Put wok back on a medium heat, adding garlic, spring onion, ginger and chilli flakes, plus 1 tbsp water if it sticks. Fry for 2 minutes, then turn up heat and add veggies: peppers, mushrooms, broccoli, and then beansprouts. Add soy, agave syrup and lemon juice. Cook for a further 4-5 minutes until vegetables are just cooked but still firm. Return tofu to the wok and gently stir through. Top with more raw beansprouts to garnish.

NB

TOFU, MADE FROM SOY BEANS, IS A LOW-FAT SOURCE OF 'COMPLETE' PROTEIN, CONTAINING ALL NINE AMINO ACIDS ESSENTIAL FOR HUMAN NUTRITION

SHORBAT RUMMAN
(Iraqi pomegranate stew)

CALORIE COUNT: 410

On a cold winter's day, this will fill you up and warm your bones – a luscious alternative to the Indian curries we all know and love. The pomegranate molasses lends further depth (it's easily sourced in supermarkets).

Serves two

2 tsps olive oil
1 large onion, diced
2 cloves, crushed
1 cinnamon stick, broken
1 tsp ground cumin
½ tsp fenugreek
pinch of saffron strands
100g yellow dried split peas
1 vegetable stock cube

1 litre vegetable stock
100g brown basmati rice
large handful of spinach, washed and chopped
2 spring onions, sliced
1 tbsp lemon juice
1 tbsp pomegranate molasses
salt and pepper
handful of coriander, chopped
handful of mint leaves, picked and chopped
pomegranate seeds

Heat oil in a large saucepan and sauté onion until softened. Add garlic and spices and cook for a further few minutes, then add split peas, stock cube and stock, and simmer for 45 minutes or until just cooked, stirring occasionally to check the stew is loose and not sticking (add further stock if so). Add rice and cook for a further 20-25 minutes, again watching consistency. Stir in spinach leaves, spring onions, lemon juice, pomegranate molasses, salt and pepper. To serve, scatter with coriander, mint and pomegranate seeds and a final twist of cracked black pepper.

NB

SPLIT PEAS ARE LOW GI AND WILL THICKEN THIS RICH STEW

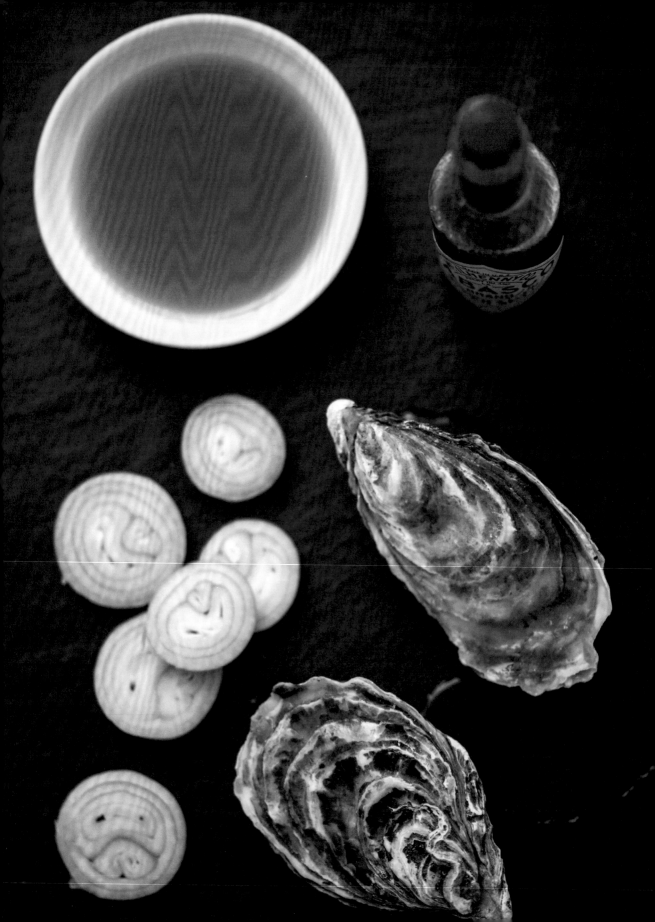

fish

OYSTERS WITH MIGNONETTE

CALORIE COUNT: 53

Oysters are thoroughly nutritious and healthy; stick to the September-April season and discard any shells that are open, cracked or damaged. Our island 'natives', farmed around Colchester and Whitstable, outrank the larger types, though they can be more expensive. The traditional accompaniment is mignonette, which in rough translation means 'cute, small, and tasty'. Precisely.

6 fresh oysters, opened

For the mignonette:
50ml white wine vinegar
50ml rice or red wine vinegar
2-3 shallots, very finely minced
¼ tsp sugar
¼ tsp salt
1 tsp ground white peppercorns
Tabasco to taste

Place mignonette ingredients in a glass bowl and stir with a fork. Cover and chill for a minimum of 4 hours, or make it a day ahead to allow the shallots to mellow in the acid of the vinegar. It will keep for 2 weeks or more in the fridge. Perhaps add a dash of Tabasco to taste.

NB

OYSTERS ARE A GREAT SOURCE OF ZINC WHICH BOOSTS THE IMMUNE SYSTEM, HEALS WOUNDS AND AIDS FERTILITY

ROAST MONKFISH WITH FENNEL, GARLIC AND ROSEMARY

CALORIE COUNT: **118** OR **133** WITH BROCCOLI

One ugly fish – flat head, mottled skin, those weird whiskery filaments – but monkfish has much to recommend it. Chefs love it for its firm meat that can cope with strong additional flavours such as the garlic, fennel and rosemary here (or, if you prefer, paprika and prosciutto or chorizo). Once the head has been removed, the rest of the fish is the 'tail' – boneless and chunky. Discard the pink membrane, which is tough once cooked, and steep it in your chosen flavours, but do make it an occasional treat; stocks are dwindling. Choose fish which are net-caught and above the size of maturity (about 70cm) from the southwest stock or from Iceland. Otherwise, swap for John Dory, red mullet or gilthead bream, all of which will more than rise to the occasion.

Serves two

2 medium-sized monkfish tails, skinless with any membrane
   removed, or other chosen fish, approximately 300g
2 garlic cloves, peeled and thinly sliced
salt and pepper
1 tsp olive oil
½ fennel bulb, thinly sliced
3 sprigs of rosemary
generous handful of curly parsley, chopped
lemon wedges to serve

Preheat the oven to 200°C/400°F. Slash the monkfish with a small, sharp knife and insert garlic slivers into the grooves. Season well. Place fennel and rosemary sprigs in a lightly oiled roasting tin, and top with the fish. Roast uncovered for 15-20 minutes until fish and fennel are cooked through. Serve with plenty of chopped parsley and lemon wedges. A pile of steamed tenderstem broccoli would be a good accompaniment.

NB

GARLIC IS WORTH ADDING TO ANY DISH – ITS ACTIVE INGREDIENT, ALLICIN, HELPS LOWER BLOOD PRESSURE, PROTECT CELLS AND REDUCE FATTY DEPOSITS[20]

GARLIC MASALA PRAWNS

CALORIE COUNT: 118

This recipe cleverly dodges the obvious 'where's the garlic butter' question; instead, it imparts kicking flavour with the spices. There's just a bit of butter, though, which adds its familiar comforting flavour. When choosing warm-water prawns, such as king and tiger, buy organic ones from a certified fishery. You may want to devein them before cooking, by peeling away the shell and slicing along the back with a small, sharp knife to remove the black filaments.

Serves two

For the masala paste:
2 tsps cumin seeds
½ cinnamon stick, broken
3 cloves
1 garlic clove, peeled and crushed
salt and pepper
2 tsps chilli powder
1 tsp ground turmeric
1 tbsp vegetable oil

To cook the prawns:
2 tsps butter
150g raw tiger prawns, shelled
juice of a lemon
handful of coriander leaves, chopped

Start with the masala paste. Heat a pan and add cumin seeds, cinnamon and cloves, dry-frying for a minute. Remove from the heat and crush in a pestle and mortar. Put this mix in a blender with garlic, salt and pepper, chilli powder, turmeric and vegetable oil and whizz to a paste. Add a splash of water if too thick. Next, melt the butter in a heavy pan, add the paste and fry for two minutes. Add the prawns and stir gently until pink, sticky and cooked through. Top with lemon juice and coriander. Serve with plenty of wilted spinach or a salad of lemon-dressed herb leaves.

NB

PRAWNS DO CONTAIN CHOLESTEROL, BUT THIS DIETARY TYPE DOES NOT IMPACT SIGNIFICANTLY ON LEVELS OF CHOLESTEROL IN THE BLOOD

CEVICHE WITH CORIANDER SALAD

CALORIE COUNT: 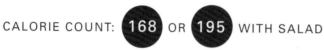 168 OR 195 WITH SALAD

If raw fish leaves you cold, try ceviche. The acid in the citrus will 'cook' the fish without heat, turning it from translucent to opalescent as you watch. This is a traditional Latin American method, and it requires, of course, the freshest fish you can muster. It works with bass, cod, mackerel – and it is particularly good with snapper. Scallops are good, too, if very fresh and plump. Serve scallops with tarragon, dill, chives or parsley instead of coriander salad.

For the ceviche:
150g red snapper fillet (or preferred fish),
   very fresh, boned, skinned and cut into 2cm cubes
juice of a lime
juice of a lemon
½ red onion, diced
½ tsp root ginger, peeled and grated
1 red chilli, deseeded and finely chopped
salt and pepper
Tabasco to taste

For the salad:
handful of herby salad leaves
1 ripe tomato, chopped
plenty of coriander, chopped

Place all the ceviche ingredients in a non-reactive bowl. Leave to marinate until the citrus has 'cooked' the fish – an hour or more. Serve with herb salad leaves, chopped tomato and coriander.

N B

UNUSUALLY FOR A 'WHITE' LOW-FAT FISH, RED SNAPPER CONTAINS A REASONABLE AMOUNT OF VITAMIN D

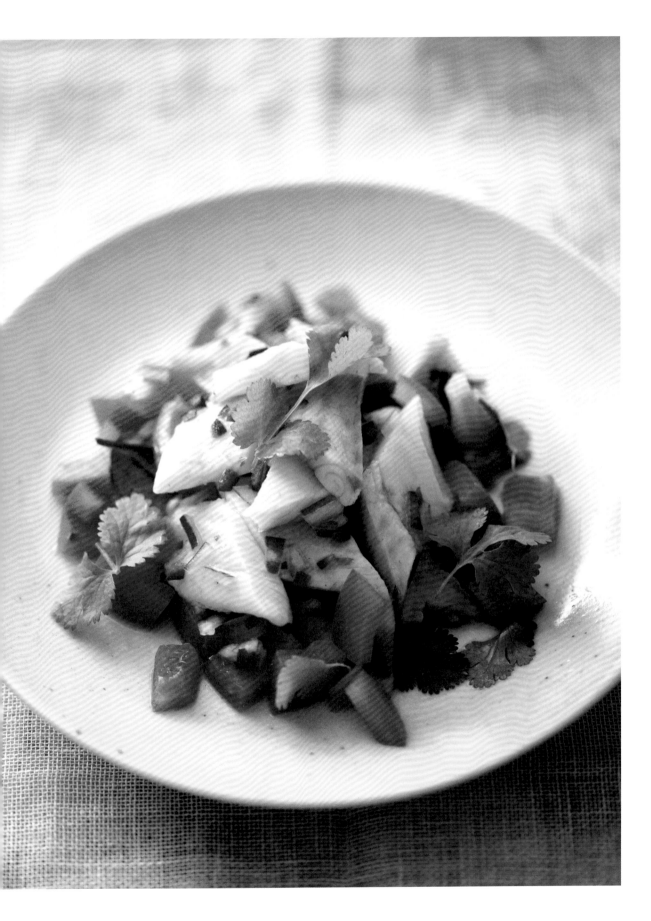

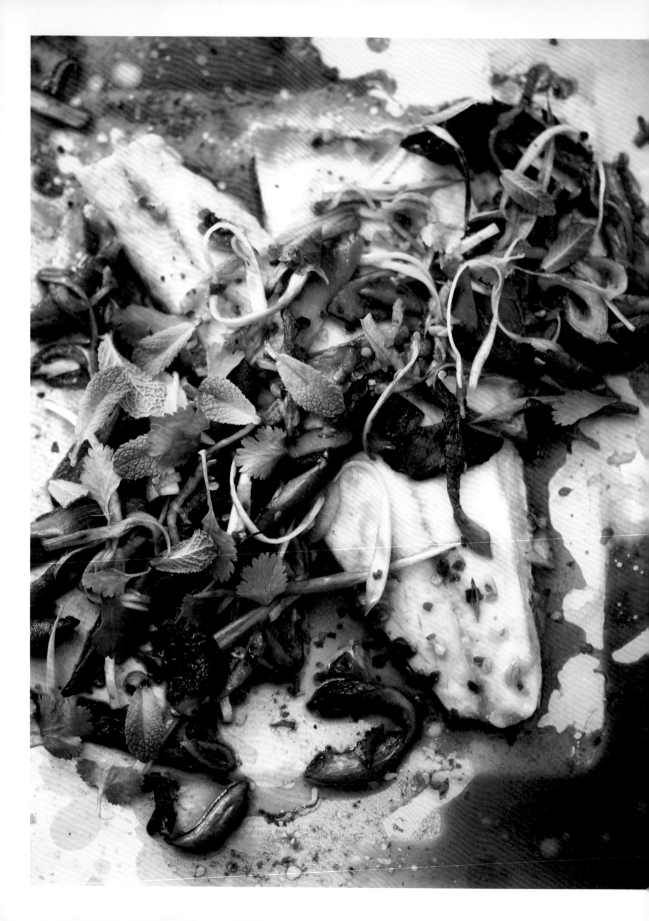

VIETNAMESE SEA BASS

CALORIE COUNT: **185**

Note the delightfully minuscule calorie count. Note the fragrant aroma as it arrives on your plate, as if from heaven itself. Poetic? Well, it is.

Serves two

2 tsps sesame oil
30g shiitake mushrooms, sliced
30g oyster mushrooms, sliced
salt and pepper
1 spring onion, julienned lengthways
½ tsp chilli flakes, or more to taste
1cm root ginger, thinly sliced
1 sea bass fillet (preferably line-caught)
1 tbsp oyster sauce
juice of half a lime
½ tbsp soy sauce
1½ tsps fish sauce
fresh herbs to garnish

Preheat the oven to 190˚C/375˚F. Heat oil in a pan, add mushrooms and season. Cook until tender – around 4-5 minutes – then combine with the spring onion, chilli and ginger. Place the sea bass in a small, ovenproof dish and add the mushroom mixture. Mix oyster sauce, lime juice, soy and fish sauces. Pour over the fish, season, and cook uncovered for 10-15 minutes. Serve scattered with fresh herbs.

WHOLE BAKED SEA BASS WITH LEMONGRASS

CALORIE COUNT: **196**

Delicate, aromatic, elegant, and – dare I say – so much easier than dialling for pizza.

Serves two

1 whole line-caught sea bass, gutted and clean (approx 500g)
3 lemongrass stems, outer leaves removed and inner stalk sliced diagonally
3cm root ginger, sliced into fine strips
2 small chillies, chopped
1 garlic clove, peeled and crushed
1 tsp honey
juice and zest of 1 lime
1 tbsp olive oil
salt and pepper

Preheat the oven to 200°C/400°F. Score the fish skin and lay whole fish on a large piece of oiled foil. Pound lemongrass in a mortar with the ginger, chilli, garlic, honey, lime juice and zest and the olive oil. Season the fish with salt and pepper, and then rub with the lemongrass mixture, inside and out and working well into the scored skin. Wrap in foil to make a loose parcel and bake for 25 minutes. Rest for a minute before opening. Alternatively, try this with lemon, flat-leaf parsley and thinly sliced fennel. *See picture, right*

NB

LEMONGRASS CONTAINS FOLATES, MINERALS AND ANTIOXIDANT VITAMINS

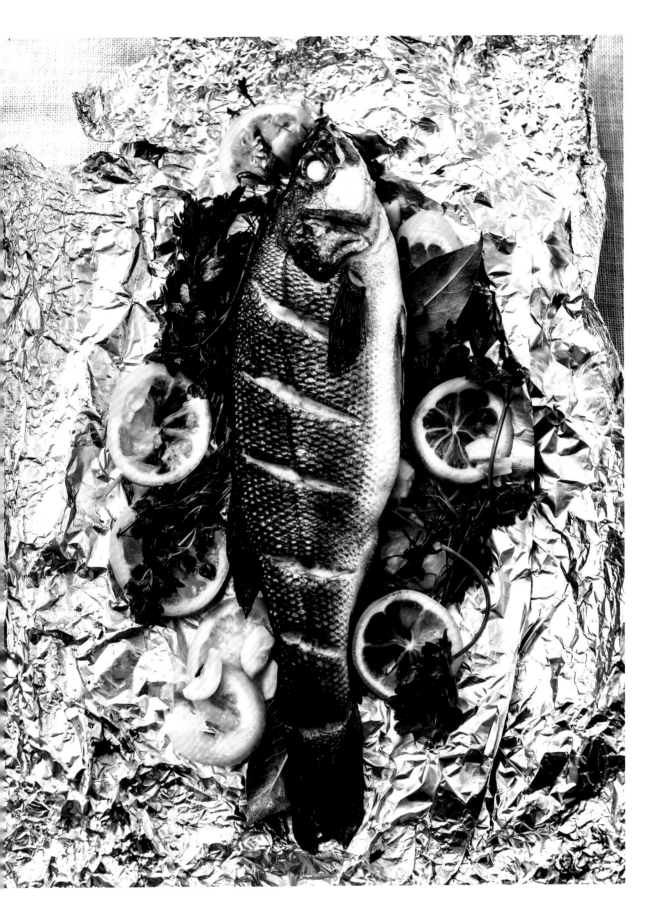

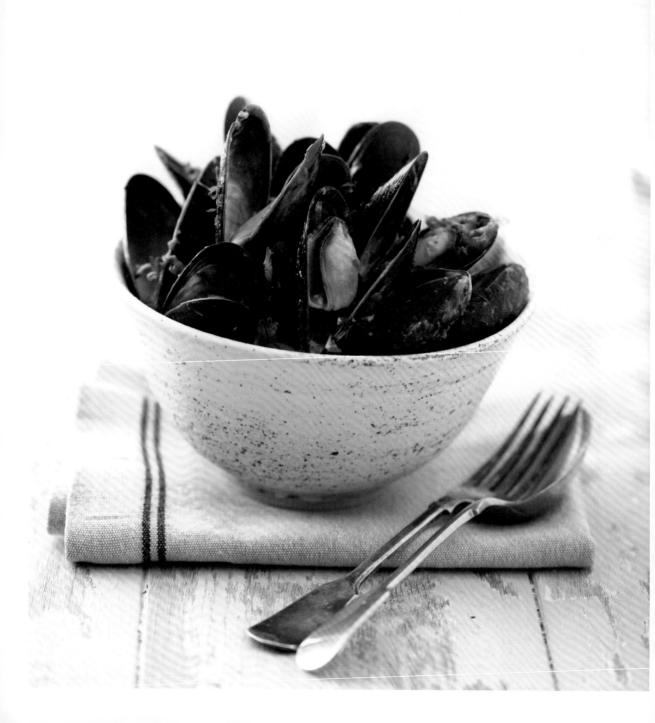

STEAMED MUSSELS IN A LIGHT TOMATO BROTH

CALORIE COUNT: **208**

Fiddly food is a bit of a bonus on a Fast Day, and mussels are a great way to get more minerals into your diet. They remain one of the most environmentally sound fish or shellfish available, though look for them in the colder months outside the breeding season, and select only those with tightly closed shells. Their plump flesh, quickly steamed in this light tomato broth, makes for an elegant little supper.

Serves four

1 tsp olive oil
2 garlic cloves, peeled and finely chopped
350g ripe tomatoes, deseeded and finely chopped
300ml fish or vegetable stock
1kg rope-grown mussels, cleaned
salt and pepper
handful of fresh parsley, chopped

Warm the oil over a medium heat in a saucepan with a tight-fitting lid. Add the garlic and cook gently for 2 minutes. Add the tomatoes and turn up the heat, cooking for a further few minutes. Add the stock and bring to the boil. Then add the mussels. Cover firmly and steam gently, shaking the pan occasionally, for 3-4 minutes, until the mussels have opened. Discard any that haven't. Season and serve in a deep soup bowl with the tomato broth, topped with fresh parsley.

NB

GRAM FOR GRAM, MUSSELS CONTAIN DOUBLE THE IRON OF RED MEAT

SMOKED HADDOCK WITH SPINACH AND POACHED EGG

CALORIE COUNT: **211**

There are few combinations as comforting as this medley – a melody, almost – of smoky fish, dark-green spinach and a quivering poached egg. It's a collaboration of flavours I well remember from childhood: a trad not a rad dish, but all the better for it. And the calories? Diddly-squat.

100g baby spinach leaves
salt and pepper
pinch of nutmeg
75g skinless smoked haddock fillet, undyed
240ml semi-skimmed milk
1 egg
1 tbsp half-fat crème fraîche
½ spring onion, finely chopped
squeeze of lemon

Wilt the spinach leaves in a little salted boiling water and drain well. Stir in a pinch of nutmeg and season. Poach the fish for 10 minutes in milk (or microwave for 3 minutes in a covered dish). Meanwhile, poach the egg (see page 24). Serve the fish and spinach topped with egg and crème fraîche mixed with spring onion and a squeeze of lemon.

This combination of ingredients also works well baked in a ramekin.
Preheat the oven to 200°C/400°F. Place a ramekin on a baking sheet. Wilt the spinach and drain well, pressing to squeeze out the moisture. Poach the fish as above until opaque, and flake with a fork. Place the spinach, fish, crème fraîche, spring onion and seasoning in a bowl and mix. Transfer to the ramekin, cover lightly with oiled foil and bake for 10-15 minutes, then remove foil, make a well in the centre of the mixture and break an egg into it. Season and bake for a further 5-8 minutes, according to how set you like your egg.

NB

COOKED SPINACH SUPPLIES MORE ANTIOXIDANTS, SUCH AS CAROTENOIDS AND FERULIC ACID, THAN RAW [21]

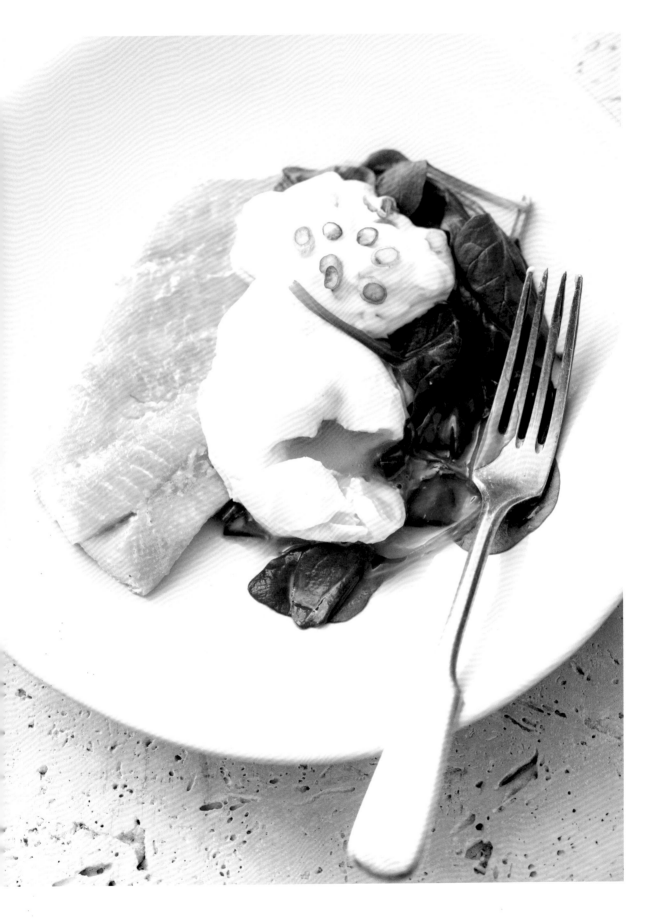

RIVER COTTAGE BREAM PARCELS IN ASIAN SPICES

CALORIE COUNT: 215

Our friend Hugh Fearnley-Whittingstall is something of a Fast Day fan, having lost 5kg in the month following Christmas. Here, then, is the kind of thing he might rustle up for a Fast Day supper. 'Baking fish scrunched up in a foil parcel with a handful of aromatics is an easy and delicious option,' says Hugh. 'Fillets of bream, gurnard, lemon sole, mullet and line-caught bass all respond well to this treatment, as well as thick fillets of pollock. And it's not just fillets that benefit from the foil parcel approach. In fact, this is one of my favourite ways to cook small-to-medium fish.'

Serves two

1 tbsp groundnut oil

2 fennel bulbs, trimmed, quartered and sliced fairly finely (2-3mm)

2 garlic cloves, peeled and finely sliced

1 tsp finely chopped root ginger

1 small red chilli, deseeded and finely sliced

2 large (150-200g) or 4 small (80-120g) fish fillets

2 tsps soy sauce

salt and pepper

Preheat oven to 190°C/375°F. Heat half the oil in a pan, add the fennel and cook gently for a few minutes. Add garlic, ginger and chilli and cook for a few minutes more, so everything starts to soften and release its flavour. Remove from heat and set aside. Take 2 pieces of strong kitchen foil, roughly 25cm square, and oil well with remaining oil. Pile the fennel mixture in the middle of each one. Season the fish fillets generously and curl around the fennel mixture – either 2 small fillets or 1 large per parcel. Sprinkle with a little soy sauce and black pepper, then bring up the sides of the foil and scrunch together tightly to form well-sealed but baggy parcels. Place on a baking tray, and bake for 15 minutes. Open up the steaming, fragrant parcels and pile the contents, including all the lovely juices, on to warm plates. Serve with wilted greens (200g), such as spinach, pak choi or choi sum.

NB

STEAMING 'EN PAPILLOTE' SEALS IN FLAVOUR AND REQUIRES VERY LITTLE ADDED FAT

LEEKS AND LEMON PRAWNS

CALORIE COUNT: **225**

A favourite quick supper at my sister-in-law Clara's house – one of those eat-from-the-bowl winners that takes the sweat out of cooking.

Serves two

2 leeks, washed and sliced into 3cm chunks
2cm root ginger, grated
¼ red chilli
1 garlic clove, peeled and crushed
juice of a lemon
1½ tsps olive oil
100g prawns, raw or pre-cooked
salt and pepper
plenty of fresh coriander, chopped

Place leeks in a steamer and cook for 4-5 minutes until tender. Combine ginger, chilli, garlic and lemon juice in a mini blender (or chop finely by hand). Sauté in olive oil for a couple of minutes before adding the prawns. Cook until prawns are fully heated or done to your liking. Add the leeks to the pan, mix through. Season, sprinkle with coriander and serve.

NB

LEEKS ARE LOW IN CALORIES (22 PER 100G) AND LOW GI TOO

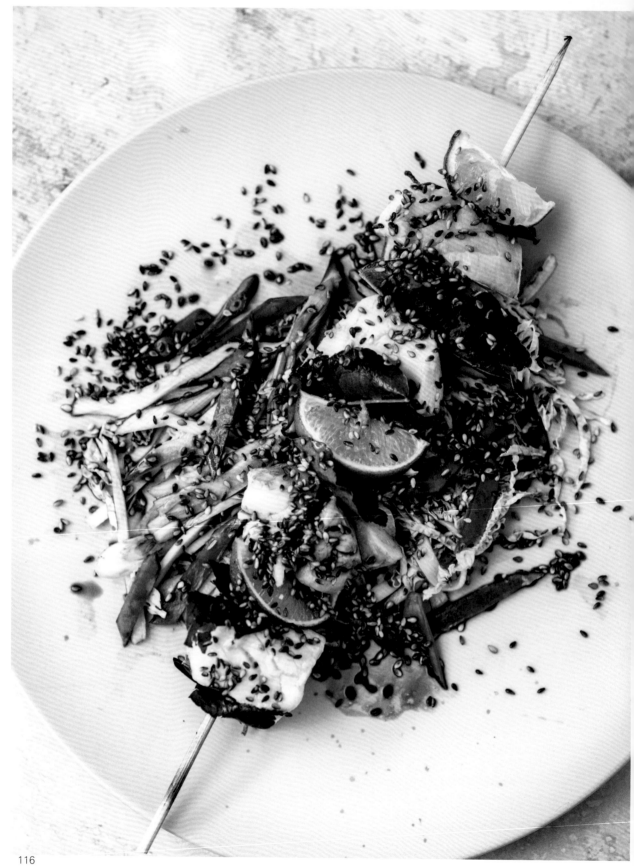

SKEWERED MONKFISH TAIL WITH BALSAMIC COLESLAW

CALORIE COUNT: **226**

These chunky, funky fish skewers will work well on a barbecue too (give them a little spray with oil before they go on the coals to stop them sticking). The lime will swell, buckle and burst in the heat, while the crisp chilli-balsamic coleslaw makes for the perfect partnership. Works with prawns too, of course.

1 tbsp lime juice
salt and pepper
1 garlic clove, crushed
150g monkfish tail, cut into thick
    chunks
kaffir lime leaves
lime wedges
groundnut oil for spraying
1-2 wooden skewers

For the coleslaw:
50g Chinese cabbage, sliced
50g mangetouts, blanched
    in boiling water, drained and
    refreshed in cold water, sliced
50g sugar snap peas, blanched as
    above, sliced
1 spring onion, finely sliced
    lengthways

For the dressing:
1 tbsp soy sauce
1½ tsps balsamic vinegar
1 tsp lime juice
1½ tsps sesame oil
1 tsp chilli flakes
1 tbsp toasted sesame seeds

Marinate the fish in the lime juice, salt, pepper and garlic and allow to rest while you prepare the coleslaw and dressing. Combine the mangetouts and sugar snap peas with the sliced cabbage and spring onion. For the dressing, mix soy sauce, vinegar, lime juice, sesame oil and chilli flakes in a small bowl. Now skewer the monkfish pieces, alternating fish with a lime wedge and a kaffir lime leaf. Heat a frying pan until hot, spray with oil and fry the skewered fish for 2 minutes on each of the 4 sides. Dress the slaw, garnish with sesame seeds, and top with fish skewers.

NB

EATING CRUCIFEROUS VEGETABLES – INCLUDING ALL KINDS OF CABBAGE – CAN HELP GUARD AGAINST CANCER[22]

STIR-FRY LEMONGRASS PRAWNS WITH MIRACLE NOODLES

CALORIE COUNT: **230**

Committed Fast Dieters will already know all about shirataki noodles. Made from a water-soluble fibre, they boast no carbs, have virtually no calories and take no time at all to prepare. That said, they taste of nothing in particular, so here lemongrass and ginger do their mighty work.

1½ tsps sesame oil
½ garlic clove, peeled and crushed
½ lemongrass stem, outer leaves removed and inner stalk finely chopped
½ red chilli, finely chopped
1 tsp root ginger, peeled and grated
1 kaffir lime leaf, shredded
6 tiger prawns, raw and shell on
1½ tsps Thai fish sauce
1 tbsp soy sauce
2 tsps lime juice
30g beansprouts
100g shirataki Miracle noodles
10g/1 tbsp unsalted peanuts, chopped
coriander leaves and lime to garnish

Heat sesame oil in a pan, and fry garlic, lemongrass, chilli and ginger until soft. Add lime leaf and 50ml water. Simmer for 5 minutes, then add prawns, fish sauce, soy sauce, lime juice and beansprouts. Cook till prawns are pink. Rinse noodles in warm water as instructions and add to prawn mix. Serve with lime wedges, torn coriander and peanuts.

NB

SHIRATAKI NOODLES ARE MADE FROM FATLESS WATER-SOLUBLE FIBRE: GLUTEN-FREE, ZERO CARBS, ZERO CALS

ALLEGRA MCEVEDY'S SCALLOPS WITH ASPARAGUS

CALORIE COUNT: **256**

Allegra, a brilliant cook and a dear mate, says: 'At the height of the season, I try to have asparagus at least three times a week, and it always feels like a treat... The dark-green leaves of the garlic plant come into season around the same time as asparagus – use baby spinach if you can't find garlic leaves, but do try to hunt them down as they are a whole new kind of fabulous.'

Serves six

100ml extra virgin olive oil
2 garlic cloves
2 bunches asparagus (allow 3-6 spears each)

1 tbsp each: chopped mint, dill, basil, chervil
squeeze of lemon
12-18 scallops (allow 2-3 per person), cleaned, keeping the rounded half of the shells

150g garlic leaves, cut into 3cm lengths, or baby spinach
salt and pepper

Preheat grill and place a rack over a foiled baking tray on the highest shelf. In a small pan, heat olive oil and garlic cloves very gently for 5-7 minutes. Slice the asparagus stalks on the diagonal into 3-4cm lengths, keeping the tips whole. Leave the garlic oil to cool to room temperature, then fish out garlic and chuck it. Once completely cool (very important, otherwise the herbs will discolour), stir in chopped herbs, a squeeze of lemon and seasoning.

Pat the scallops dry and season well. Put a wide-bottomed pan on a high heat with about 150ml water. Bring to the boil and add asparagus. Cover and steam for 2 minutes.

Place scallops (not touching) on the hot rack and stick it back under the grill. They will take 2-4 minutes on each side depending on size.

Take the lid off the asparagus pot and add garlic leaves or spinach. Shake it – the idea is that the greens are just wilted as all the water evaporates. Check the scallops are cooked (opaque with a small amount of resistance when you squeeze them round the middle). Add two thirds of the soft herb dressing to the pan with the greens and toss well. Divide greens between the shells or small plates and top with the scallops. To finish, drizzle generously with the remaining herb dressing.

SALMON FILLET THREE WAYS

Broken, with cucumber and dill

CALORIE COUNT: **257**

1 salmon fillet (100g)
salt and pepper
50g round lettuce, leaves washed and dried
50g cos leaves, washed and dried
50g baby spinach
¼ cucumber, quartered, seeds removed and sliced

For the dressing:
2 tbsps low-fat yoghurt
juice of half a lime
handful of fresh dill

Season the salmon and steam until opaque. Set aside to cool. Mix the dressing ingredients. Put leaves and cucumber on a plate and break the warm salmon into pieces on top. Dress and garnish with more dill and lime wedges.

O'Kelly fish

CALORIE COUNT: **318**

Serves four

400g trimmed green beans, blanched and refreshed
200g broccoli florets, blanched and refreshed
200g asparagus spears, blanched and refreshed
juice of 2 lemons, plus husks
2 tbsps olive oil
1 tsp chilli flakes
salt and pepper
30g black Greek olives
4 vines of cherry tomatoes, vine included
4 salmon fillets (100g each)

Preheat oven to 200°C/400°F. Place blanched veggies and seasonings in a large roasting pan, squeezing the juice of 1 lemon over them. Drizzle with olive oil. Scatter in the olives and place vine tomatoes on top. Lay the fillets, skin side down, as a top layer, and squeeze over the second lemon, throwing in the husks. Oven roast for 20 minutes. The tomatoes and lemon will have made a wonderful juice to spoon over the fish. *See picture, right*

Poached, with greens and a tomato-anchovy dressing

CALORIE COUNT: **321**

½ fennel bulb, thinly sliced
salt and pepper
1 bay leaf
1 salmon fillet (100g)
100g green beans, steamed but still al dente
100g sugar snap peas, also lightly steamed

For the dressing and garnish:
1 ripe tomato, finely chopped
1 anchovy fillet, finely chopped
1 spring onion, finely chopped
1 tbsp lemon juice
2 tsps olive oil
handful of torn basil leaves

Bring a pan of water to the boil, add the fennel, salt and pepper and bay leaf and boil for 5 minutes. Remove from heat. Add the salmon, cover and set aside for 15 minutes. Remove the fish and break into bite-sized chunks. Serve on the steamed beans and sugar snaps, along with a little fennel from the pan. Drizzle with dressing and top with torn basil leaves.

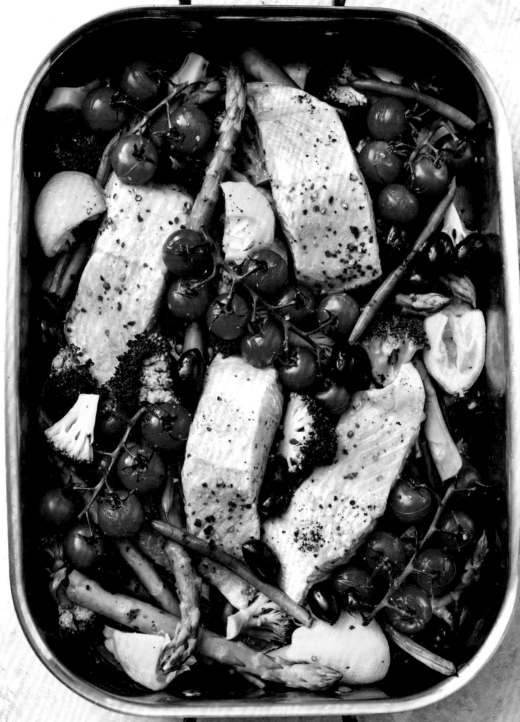

WHITE FISH STEW WITH ORANGE AND FENNEL

CALORIE COUNT: **268**

Greek legend has it that a fennel stalk carried the coal that passed down knowledge from the gods to men. I couldn't possibly say, but I do know that this marriage of fennel, firm fish and zingy orange verges on the divine.

Serves four

For the fish stock:
500g fish offcuts (no oily fish) plus any bones
1 onion, quartered
1 celery stalk
trimmings of fennel bulb (see stew ingredients, right)
1 tbsp peppercorns

For the stew:
2 tbsps olive oil
1 onion, thinly sliced
3 garlic cloves, thinly sliced
1 small fennel bulb, thinly sliced
1 tsp coriander seeds
250ml fish stock
1 orange – juice and 2 strips of peel
1 400g tin chopped tomatoes
2 bay leaves

½ tsp herbes de Provence or tarragon
pinch of saffron
salt and pepper
750g white fish fillet, such as pollock, monkfish or halibut
8 tiger prawns, shells on
fresh parsley

To make your own stock, put fish offcuts (if buying filleted fish, ask for the bones – you can freeze them for later use) in a deep pan. Add the onion, celery, fennel trimmings and peppercorns and cover with water. Simmer for about 45 minutes and strain, removing any froth.

For the stew, heat oil in a large non-stick saucepan and gently fry the onion, fennel, garlic and coriander seeds for 15 minutes, until tender. Add fish stock, orange juice, orange peel and tomatoes, and add a tomato tin of cold water. Add bay leaves, herbs and saffron. Season and simmer for 20-25 minutes. Add fish, monkfish first if using, prawns last. Cover and cook for a further 4 minutes until fish and prawns are cooked through. Serve piping hot and scattered with fresh parsley.

NB

A GOOD STOCK IS THE BACKBONE HERE – FULL OF MINERALS, FULL OF FLAVOUR

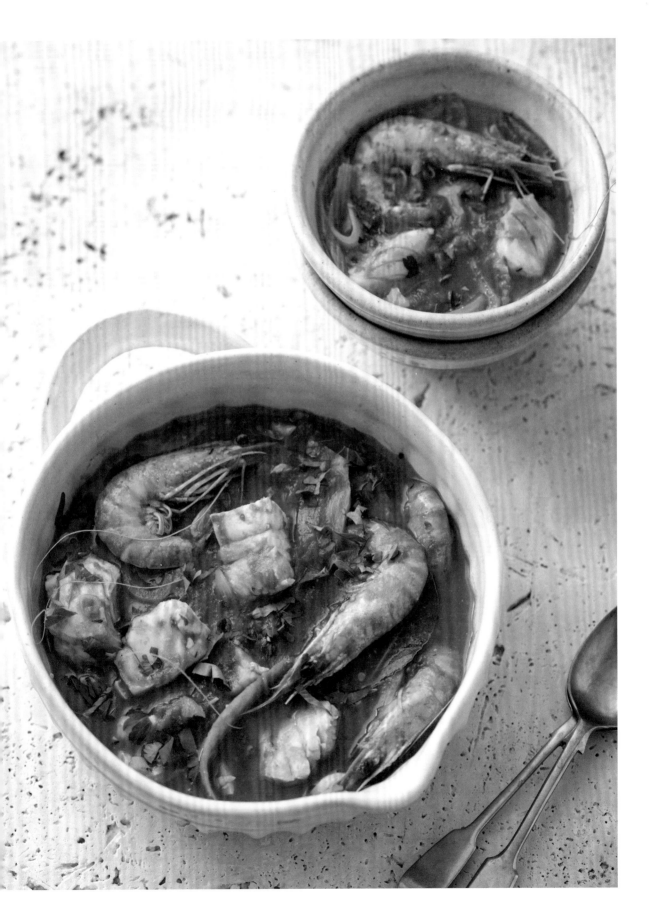

TUNA FAGIOLI

CALORIE COUNT: **286**

This is one of the quick and tasty Italian dishes I grew up on, and today it makes the perfect Fast Day supper – comfortably low in all the things you ought to avoid, but sky-high in flavour. It is simplicity itself to prepare, a real store-cupboard stand-by, and – like chilli con carne – it tastes even better the following day. You could drain the tuna to save on calories, though you'd need to replace it with olive oil if you do; some oil is essential here. But don't panic. Not much.

Serves two

1 100g tin tuna in olive oil, undrained
400g tinned beans, drained – choose from kidney,
   haricot, cannellini, garbanzo or butter beans
½ red onion, thinly sliced or chopped
1 tbsp white wine vinegar
juice of half a lemon
1 garlic clove, peeled and crushed
2 fat ripe tomatoes, sliced
flat-leaf parsley, torn
rock salt and freshly ground pepper

Put everything except the tomatoes and parsley in a bowl. Mix and leave to settle for 30 minutes. Serve with sliced tomatoes generously sprinkled with parsley, rock salt and freshly ground pepper.

NB

THE BENEFICIAL SULPHUR COMPOUNDS IN ONIONS CAN BE DESTROYED IN COOKING; HERE, RAW RED ONION IS LESS AGGRESSIVE THAN WHITE

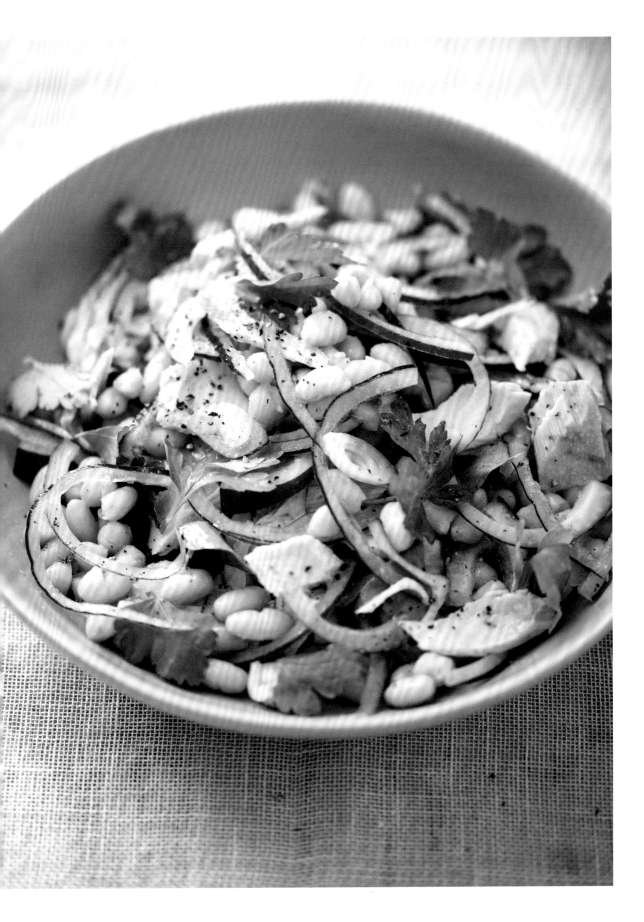

SEARED SESAME TUNA FOUR WAYS

CALORIE COUNT: **317**

This recipe uses tuna loin, which ought to be eaten rare. That way, it melts in the mouth and is a real treat to eat. Tuna is oil-rich and provides a great source of lean protein, but buy it and eat it with care. The NHS and FSL recommend limiting consumption of certain fish because they may contain environmental pollutants; one serving of tuna a week is the current quota. As far as sustainability goes, look for pole-and-line skipjack from the Maldives or Albacore from the Pacific, and check that your tuna has been caught using 'dolphin-friendly' methods.

200g fresh tuna loin
1 tsp olive oil
salt and pepper
2 tsps sesame seeds

Heat a griddle pan until very hot. Rub the tuna with olive oil and season well. Roll it in the sesame seeds. Cook on each side for 30 seconds, leaving the interior as rare as you dare.

With soy-mirin dressing

CALORIE COUNT: ADD (19)

Make a dressing from 1 tbsp mirin, 1 tbsp soy sauce and 1 tbsp rice wine vinegar. Top the sliced seared tuna with 50g shredded daikon, 50g julienned cucumber and a handful each of mint leaves and coriander. Drizzle with dressing.

With lemongrass dipping sauce

CALORIE COUNT: ADD (28)

Combine 1 tbsp Thai fish sauce, 1 tbsp lime juice, ½ tsp brown sugar, ½ stem finely chopped lemongrass, ½ sliced red chilli, ½ chopped garlic clove. Spoon over sliced tuna. This dip works well with other fish too. Try it with king prawns, lemon sole or net-trawled Dover sole, if you want to tick the sustainable boxes. Sole has a low oil content, so cook it quickly to avoid drying it out.

With chilli green beans

CALORIE COUNT: ADD (50)

Heat a little sesame oil and fry a chopped shallot, 1 tsp nigella or fennel seeds and ½ tsp chilli flakes. Add a handful of blanched thin green beans (50g) and ½ tbsp oyster sauce. Cook till beans are tender.

With salsa verde

CALORIE COUNT: ADD (121)

Make enough salsa for 4 servings (it will keep in the fridge for 4-5 days) from 1 tsp Dijon mustard, 50ml extra virgin olive oil and the juice and zest of half a lemon. Whisk or shake to emulsify. Add 2 finely chopped anchovy fillets, a handful each of fresh flat-leaf parsley, mint, basil and tarragon, all chopped, and 1 tsp chopped rinsed capers. Crush a garlic clove to a paste with sea salt and add. Mix well, and drizzle over the sliced tuna.

NB

NB ONLY FRESH TUNA COUNTS TOWARDS OILY FISH INTAKE; TINNED TUNA LOSES MOST OF ITS OMEGA-3 FATS DURING THE CANNING PROCESS

HERRING WITH A SPICED ALMOND CRUST

CALORIE COUNT: **350**

Ah, the underrated, overlooked herring. They throng our coastal waters, are modest, inexpensive and a fine way to get your omega-3 fix. Thames herring is certified by the Marine Stewardship Council, so eat it with abandon. Or with this nutty crust.

2 herring fillets (approximately 100g)
25g whole blanched almonds
handful flat-leaf parsley, chopped
½ tsp grated orange zest
1 garlic clove, peeled and crushed

½ tsp ground cumin
pinch of chilli flakes
salt and pepper
juice of half a lemon

Preheat oven to 180°C/350°F. Wash herring, dry and set to one side. Combine other ingredients and pulse in a processor until blended to a paste. Rub fish with paste and place in a small shallow roasting pan. Bake for 8-10 minutes until fish is cooked. Serve with plenty of lemon.

Or try rubbed with 1 tbsp shop-bought tapenade (240 calories).

Or doused with the juice of a lime, rolled in 2 tsps plain flour and seasoned with plenty of cracked black pepper and sea salt (246 calories).

Or with a honey-mustard crust: 1 tbsp pinhead oats, 2 tsps Dijon mustard, ½ tsp honey (289 calories).

NB

HERRINGS PROVIDE HIGH-QUALITY PROTEIN AND GOOD FATS FOR LITTLE COST

ALLEGRA MCEVEDY'S BAKE-IN-THE BAG FISH WITH PRESERVED LEMON COUSCOUS

CALORIE COUNT: **364**

Says Allegra: 'This is just about the healthiest and easiest supper I know. It's an all-in-one, steam-in-the-bag number, which lets the flavours just hang out and party together without getting busted. The real joy of this is what happens to the couscous, which cooks in the fish juices and greedily absorbs all the aromatics. If you can't get monkfish, any fresh, white fish will do. The bags can be made up a few hours ahead of time and kept in the fridge.'

Serves six

250g couscous
2 tsps ground cumin
1 tsp cumin seeds
6 spring onions, thinly sliced

2 preserved lemons, roughly
   chopped
10g coriander, roughly chopped
18 cherry tomatoes, quartered
1.2kg fish fillet – try this with
   monkfish, halibut, turbot

3 tbsps olive oil
1 tsp saffron
2 small fennel bulbs, halved,
   core removed, sliced
salt and pepper

Preheat oven to 200°C/400°F. Mix all the ingredients, except the fish, olive oil, saffron and fennel, in a bowl and season. Slice the fish fillet, allowing around 2-3 'medallions' per person. Boil 180ml water in a small pan and add saffron, then remove from heat. Coat dry couscous mixture in 2 tbsps olive oil, and pour in the saffron water. Stir. Take 6 sheets of kitchen foil and lay them out with the short side towards you. Lightly oil each sheet and place a sixth of the fennel on top. Place a neat little mound of the couscous mixture on each pile of fennel. Top with fish, drizzle with remaining olive oil, season and, as Allegra says, 'Take a few moments to see how pretty it looks.'

Fold the parcels, ensuring that all are well sealed, leaving just the tops open, then pour 3 tbsps water into each. Seal the top edge of each parcel and place on a baking tray. Bake for 15-20 minutes, until parcels have puffed up nicely. Take your little pillows out of the oven and serve straight onto warm plates, allowing your guests to eat from the foil – very little washing up!

NB

STEAMING HELPS PRESERVE WATER-SOLUBLE VITS THAT ARE ORDINARILY LOST IN BOILING

CHARRED SQUID WITH BUTTER BEANS AND CHILLI

CALORIE COUNT: **369**

A glorious collision of flavour and texture, and marvellously on-message for a Fast Day supper. It's not dirt cheap in calories, but what can I say? You get what you pay for.

200g squid, cleaned and trimmed
salt and pepper
200g (½ tin) butter beans
1 tbsp fresh parsley, chopped, plus more for serving
1½ tsps lemon juice
generous handful of rocket
1 tsp olive oil
1 red chilli, thinly sliced
squeeze of lime

Score the squid and season. Gently heat butter beans in a small saucepan, adding chopped parsley and a little of the lemon juice. Heat a griddle pan till almost smoking. Cook squid for a minute on each side, until slightly blackened here and there. Dress rocket with remaining lemon, olive oil, more salt and pepper and the red chilli. Slice squid and mix into leaves. Serve with a squeeze of lime, more fresh parsley and the seasoned butter beans.

NB

SQUID IS LOW IN SATURATED FATS. JUST DON'T BATTER AND FRY IT ON A FAST DAY…

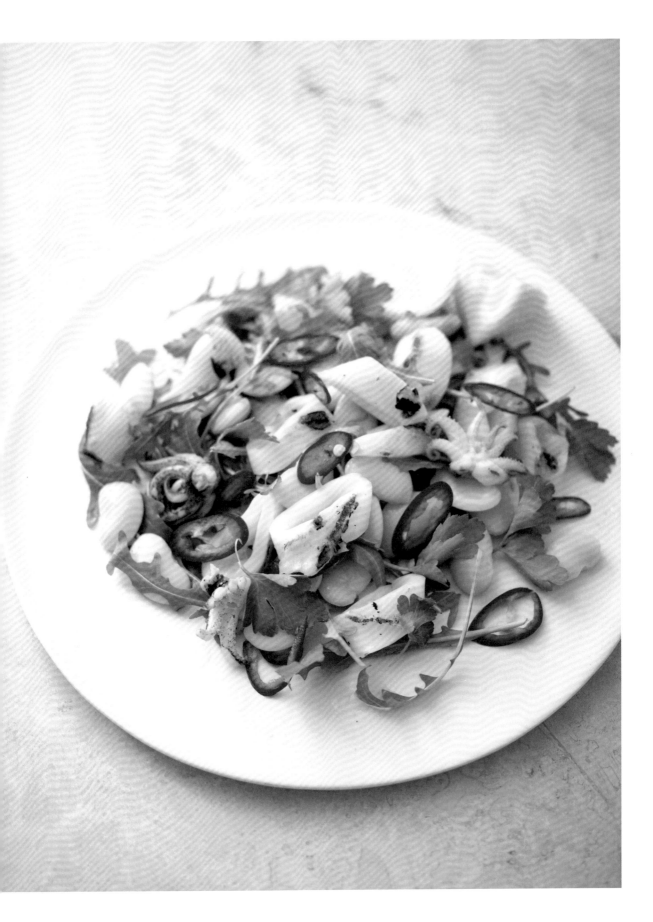

ROAST SARDINES WITH MOROCCAN SPICES

CALORIE COUNT: **399**

If you want to combine all your concerns – physiological, financial, environmental – in one fine little fish, look to Cornish sardines or pilchards: loaded with protein, high in omega 3s, cheap as chips, and impressively light in contaminants since they live low on the food chain. Go for sardines caught in traditional drift or ring nets, and be generous with the parsley.

1½ tsps cumin seeds
1½ tsps coriander seeds
2 garlic cloves
handful of fresh coriander, plus
   more for serving
handful of fresh flat-leaf parsley
cayenne pepper to taste
juice of half a lemon

1½ tsps paprika
2 tsps flaxseed oil
2 sardine fillets, gutted and
cleaned (approx 200g)
lemon wedges and red onion,
   thinly sliced, to serve

Dry-fry the cumin and coriander seeds in a frying pan, then use a pestle and mortar to grind to a powder (if in a hurry, you could use 1 tbsp garam masala instead). Blend garlic and herbs in a processor, then add ground spice mix, cayenne, paprika and lemon juice. Emulsify with the flaxseed oil. Slash the sardine skin and rub with the mixture. Leave for 2 hours in the fridge, then bake for 8-10 minutes at 200°C/400°F. Serve with fresh lemon wedges, more coriander and a scatter of thinly sliced red onion.

NB

A DIET RICH IN OMEGA-3 FATTY ACIDS – SARDINES AND MACKEREL ARE BRILLIANT SOURCES – HELPS TO CUT YOUR RISK OF HEART DISEASE AND SOME CANCERS[23]

SEARED MACKEREL ON A RAINBOW SALAD

CALORIE COUNT: **457**

Until recently, mackerel ticked all our boxes: great taste, full of beneficent oils, local to our waters, relatively cheap… The story has now become more complicated, chiefly because mackerel is being overfished. Good alternatives include herring and sardine, though if you still want to eat mackerel, look for 'handline-caught', which is considered the most sustainable.

1 mackerel fillet (100g)
salt and pepper
1 tbsp oil
½ yellow pepper and ½ red pepper, thinly sliced
½ red onion, thinly sliced
1 medium carrot, peeled and shredded

For the dressing:
1½ tsps crunchy peanut butter
5 tbsps lime juice
1 tsp Thai fish sauce
1 garlic clove, peeled and minced
2cm root ginger, grated
1 lemongrass stem, outer leaves removed
   and inner stalk finely chopped or minced
1 tsp raw agave syrup
chopped red chilli to taste
lemon wedges to serve
coriander leaves

Score the mackerel fillet and season well. Sear in a hot heavy pan with a little oil until skin is crisp. Mix the veg and place on a plate. Combine dressing ingredients. Place warm fish on the vegetable salad and serve drizzled with 1 tbsp dressing and plenty of lemon wedges and fresh coriander leaves.

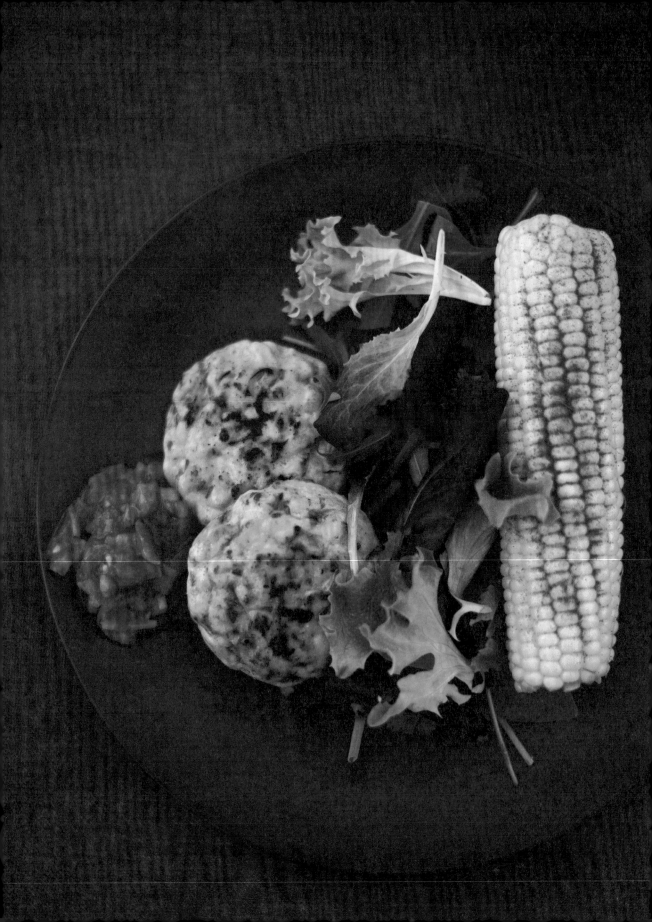

meat

CUMIN-SCENTED TURKEY BURGERS WITH TOMATO SALSA

CALORIE COUNT: **174** OR **333** WITH CORN-ON-THE-COB AND SALSA

Swapping beef for turkey will slash the calories in a burger (and, incidentally, the cost) – but you do need a little egg to bind it all together in a steady embrace, otherwise the meat is liable to dry out and will collapse before your very eyes.

125g turkey mince
1 spring onion, finely chopped
1 small egg, beaten – use about 1 tbsp
½ red chilli, deseeded and finely chopped
1 garlic clove, peeled and crushed
½ tsp ground cumin
½ tsp ground coriander
salt and pepper

To serve:
herby salad leaves
corn-on-the-cob, boiled and
   dusted with paprika
classic tomato salsa (see
   page 202)

Combine all the burger ingredients and leave to marinate for half an hour in the fridge. Shape into 2 patties and grill for 5-7 minutes on each side, until cooked through. Serve with lemon-dressed herby salad leaves, classic tomato salsa and corn-on-the-cob.

BAKED PORK TENDERLOIN WITH FENNEL

CALORIE COUNT: **220**

Fennel and pork are best of friends, and they probably converse in Italian. This is a flavourful, lip-smacking dish, full of good things for relatively little calorie expenditure.

Serves two

2 tsps fennel seeds, crushed to release flavour
salt and pepper
1 pork tenderloin, approximately 300g
oil for spraying
200ml chicken stock
2 garlic cloves, peeled and crushed
2 medium fennel bulbs, trimmed and cut into
   quarters (keep the fronds for garnish)
½ tbsp olive oil
good squeeze of lemon juice
lemon wedges to serve

Preheat oven to 180°C/350°F. Sprinkle crushed fennel seeds and seasoning onto a piece of baking parchment. Spray the pork with a little oil, then roll in the seeds and seasoning. Sear in a hot pan for a minute on each side to seal and colour the meat. Remove pork, then add stock and crushed garlic to deglaze the pan, cooking for 2 minutes until heated through and garlic is beginning to soften. Place fennel quarters in a small baking tray, add garlicky stock juices, olive oil and lemon juice; season, and place seared pork fillet on top. Bake for 15-20 minutes, covering loosely with foil if necessary to keep the meat moist.

Remove pork from oven and rest on a chopping board, returning the fennel to the oven for a final 5 minutes to further reduce remaining liquid. Slice pork into thick medallions and serve on a bed of hot fennel, drizzled with pan juices and decorated with fennel fronds and a lemon wedge or two.

GREEN PAPAYA SALAD WITH CHARGRILLED BEEF

CALORIE COUNT: **221**

Unripe or 'green' papaya is the foundation for this sparky *som tam* salad, bristling with Thai taste and chilli heat. Christopher Columbus called the papaya 'the fruit of the angels', and a shredded green one might well be the perfect raw food. The salad is oil-free too. Bingo.

For the dressing:
1 garlic clove, peeled and crushed
½ red chilli, finely chopped
1 tsp palm sugar
1 tbsp Thai fish sauce
1 tbsp lime juice

For the salad and garnish:
½ green papaya, peeled and finely
   shredded or sliced into strips
¼ cucumber, shredded
1 spring onion, sliced
handful of Thai basil leaves,
   mint leaves and coriander
100g sirloin steak
lime wedges to serve

Place garlic, chilli, palm sugar, fish sauce and lime juice in a bowl and stir. Combine the salad vegetables, and dress with the garlic mixture. Grill the steak to your liking – it's best if pink – and let it rest. Slice and serve with lime wedges on top of the dressed salad. Perhaps add a scatter of pomegranate seeds. This combination of ingredients also works well with grilled king prawns.

NB

HALF A PAPAYA PROVIDES HALF YOUR RECOMMENDED DAILY AMOUNT OF VITAMIN C

CHICKEN BREAST EIGHT WAYS

Yes, I know. Chicken is a bore. You're not supposed to order it in restaurants – everyone will yawn and the chef will mark you down as a wuss for not ordering his fricasséed sweetbreads. But. Most of us love it and we certainly eat a lot of the stuff. Chicken fillets are simple to prepare, low in calories (around 127 per fillet), quick to cook – and, when teamed with powerhouse flavours like these, you can't get a much better weekday supper, especially if you buy a fine free-range, organic bird. Be sure to remove the skin to lessen the calorie load, though if you are going to roast a chicken breast, keep the skin on until after cooking to prevent the meat drying out (the inarguable scourge of chicken dinners everywhere).

Lime chicken salad, Szechuan style

CALORIE COUNT: 195

1 small chicken breast, skin on (110g)
a little olive oil
salt and pepper
½ cucumber, sliced lengthways, deseeded and cut on
 the diagonal into crescents
handful of coriander, including finely chopped stalks
handful of mint leaves
½ tsp ground Szechuan peppercorns, crushed
1 tbsp Thai fish sauce
1 tsp sesame oil
1 spring onion, finely sliced diagonally
2 tbsps lime juice
shredded iceberg lettuce (80g)
lime wedges to serve

Preheat oven to 190°C/375°F. Oil the chicken breast lightly before seasoning with salt and pepper (skin to be removed after cooking). Bake, covered, in oven until cooked through and juices run clear – about 20 minutes. Allow to cool. Tear chicken into shreds and place in a bowl with cucumber, most of the coriander and mint. Make a dressing from the Szechuan pepper, fish sauce, sesame oil, spring onion, lime juice and seasoning. Combine with chicken mixture and serve on shredded iceberg lettuce, garnished with lime wedges and more coriander leaves.

Masala style with raita

CALORIE COUNT: **199**

OR **219** WITH SPINACH

Marinate a skinless chicken breast in juice of lemon, ½ crushed garlic clove, ½ tsp ground cumin, 1 crushed cardomom pod, 2 bruised cloves, ½ tsp fenugreek, ½ tsp ground turmeric, a pinch of cayenne, salt and pepper and 1 tsp grated root ginger. Add a squeeze of lime. Refrigerate for at least an hour, or overnight. Grill chicken for 7 minutes on each side and serve with 2 tbsps low-fat natural yoghurt combined with chopped cucumber, mint and a sprinkle of cumin seeds (or see raita recipe on page 203). This also calls for 100g wilted spinach.

Teriyaki with sesame seeds

CALORIE COUNT: **227**

Mix 1 tbsp soy sauce with 1 tbsp sake, 2 tbsps mirin, 3 tbsps water, 1 tsp grated root ginger and ½ tsp sugar. Heat ingredients and gently simmer a skinless chicken breast in the broth until poached – around 15-20 minutes. Dry-toast 1 tbsp sesame seeds until golden brown and set aside. Remove chicken from broth and allow to rest under foil. Bring broth back to the boil and reduce, stirring occasionally, until glossy and slightly sticky – about 5 minutes. Slice chicken breast and serve with sauce, sprinkled with sesame seeds. Add a good quantity of steamed pak choi.

Summer poached with lean greens

CALORIE COUNT: **252**

Bring a pan of water to the boil, adding a handful of chopped coriander stems, 3 peppercorns, 1 tsp grated root ginger, 1 roughly chopped shallot and 1 tsp rock salt. Add skinless chicken breast and simmer for 15-20 minutes until cooked through. Blanch 50g broccoli florets, 50g sugar snap peas, 50g asparagus spears and 75g young spinach leaves for a minute in boiling water and drain well on kitchen paper. Remove chicken from broth and slice. Serve on top of the cooked veg and drizzle with a dressing made from ½ tsp chili flakes, 1 tsp raw agave nectar, 1½ tsps rice vinegar, 1 tbsp lime juice, 1 tbsp fish sauce, 1 star anise, ½ tsp garlic powder, salt and pepper. Garnish with torn coriander, mint leaves and lime wedges.

Skewered Italian

CALORIE COUNT: **260**

Flatten a chicken breast by placing it between two sheets of greaseproof paper and beating lightly with rolling pin. Top with 1 chopped ripe beef tomato, a few basil leaves and 2 tsps freshly grated Parmesan. Season, roll up, skewer with a toothpick and grill under a medium heat, turning once until done. Serve with a large helping of tenderstem broccoli or some dry-griddled courgette strips.

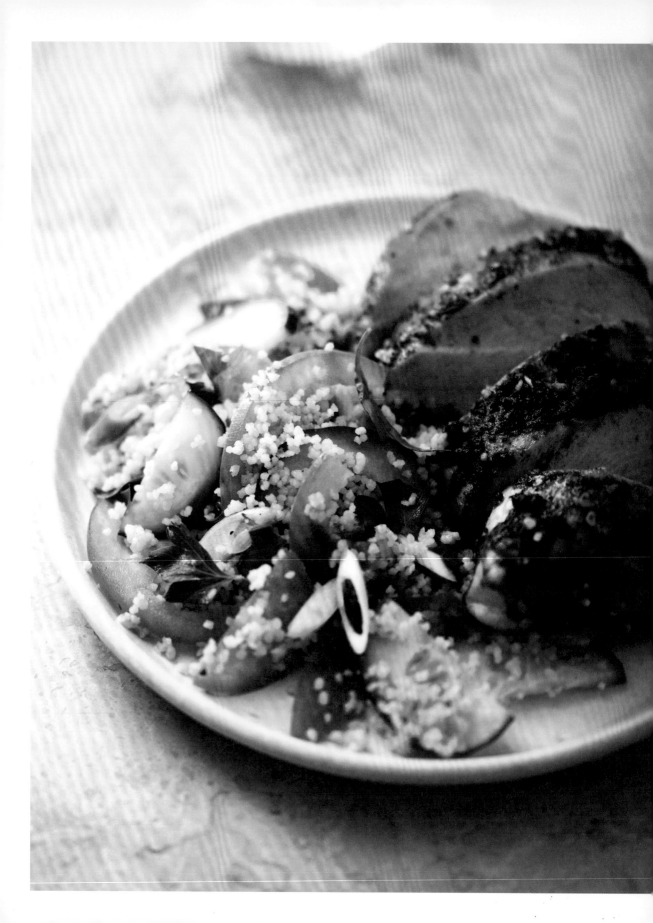

French tarragon and lemon

CALORIE COUNT: 267

Cut a skinless chicken breast into goujons, fry in 1 tsp olive oil for 5-6 minutes until golden, moving the pieces around to prevent sticking (add a little water if they do). Remove pan from heat and add 1 tbsp half-fat crème fraîche, the juice of half a lemon and a generous tbsp chopped fresh tarragon. Season and serve with 50g each of steamed mangetouts and sugar snap peas. Garnish with tarragon sprigs.

Romano peppers and spinach

CALORIE COUNT: 290

Lightly steam a skinless chicken breast for 15 minutes until cooked through. Heat 1 tsp olive oil in a pan. Slice 1 orange pepper and 1 red pepper and add to pan, together with a sprig of rosemary, the juice of half a lemon and a sliced garlic clove and sauté for 5 minutes. Add 100ml water and allow to reduce and become sticky. Add a handful of spinach leaves for the final 2 minutes of cooking, and serve with the sliced steamed chicken breast, a few sea salt flakes and a grating of fresh lemon zest.

Harissa-spiked with giant couscous

CALORIE COUNT: 300

Smear a chicken breast with 2 tsps harissa paste and drizzle with a little oil. Season. Bake in oven at 170°C/325°F for 20-25 minutes until cooked and juices run clear. Cover with foil if the edges of the chicken threaten to burn before it is cooked. Serve with 3 tbsps prepared giant couscous (simply add boiling water according to packet instructions), combined with 1 chopped spring onion, 1 chopped tomato, ¼ chopped cucumber, chopped flat-leaf parsley and mint. *See picture, left*

NB

CHICKEN PROVIDES IMPORTANT B VITAMINS, AND ITS PROTEIN AIDS SATIETY

LIGHTWEIGHT COTTAGE PIE

CALORIE COUNT: **243**

The pleasingly low calorie count here is achieved by swapping the usual topping of buttered potato mash for a lighter celeriac and leek lid, and using less meat than usual. The idea remains the same – a pot of unctuous loveliness to see you through a cold snap.

Serves four

oil for spraying
250g extra-lean minced beef
1 large onion, diced
2 carrots, peeled and diced
2 celery stalks, finely chopped
1 400g tin chopped tomatoes
2 tbsps tomato purée
1 tbsp Worcestershire sauce
1 bay leaf

1 tsp fresh thyme leaves, chopped
salt and pepper
300ml boiling water
2 Oxo cubes
500g celeriac, peeled and cubed
100g half-fat crème fraîche
1 tsp groundnut oil
2 young leeks, trimmed and
    sliced (pound-coin width)

Preheat oven to 200°C/400°F. Spray a large pan with oil and brown minced beef. Add *mirepoix* (diced onion, celery and carrot) and allow to soften for 10 minutes. Stir in chopped tomatoes, tomato purée, Worcestershire sauce, bay leaf, thyme, salt and pepper, water and Oxo cubes. Bring to the boil, cover and simmer for 30 minutes, stirring occasionally. Meanwhile, boil celeriac until very tender, drain and mash with crème fraîche until as smooth as you wish. Heat oil in a pan and gently sauté leeks, then add them to the celeriac mash; season well. Pour beef into a shallow ovenproof dish and top with celeriac mixture. Bake for 20-30 minutes, until top is golden brown.

NB

USING CELERIAC INSTEAD OF MASHED POTATO REDUCES THE CALORIES BY 75%

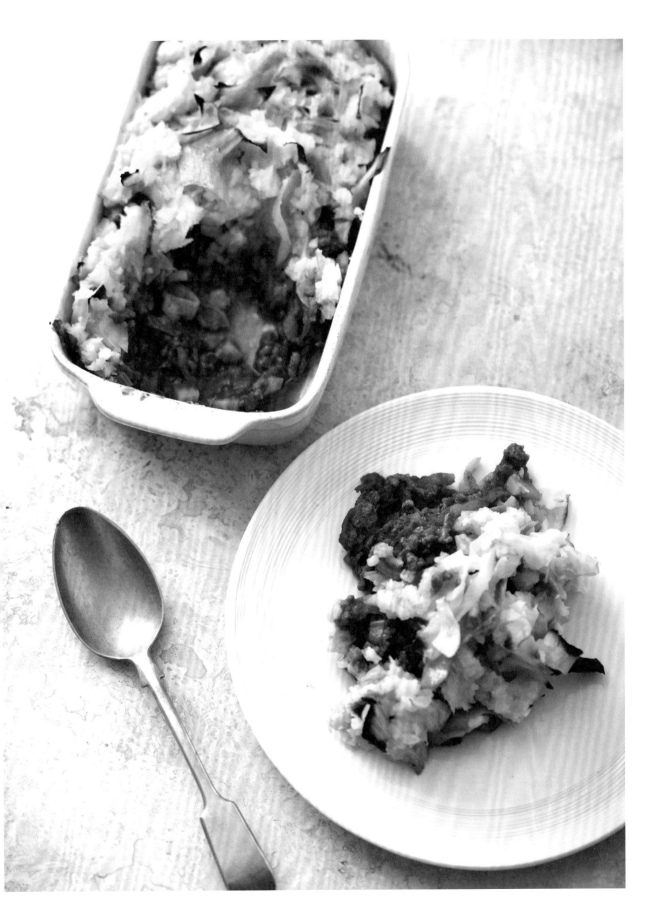

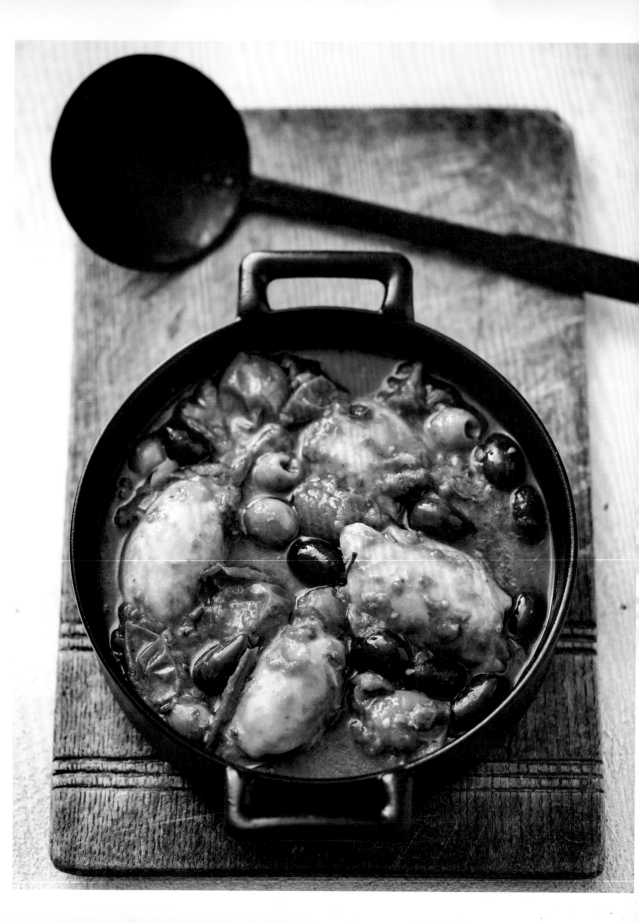

SARAH RAVEN'S CHICKEN PUTTANESCA

CALORIE COUNT: **247**

Horticulturalist, kitchen gardener and cook, Sarah Raven is also a Fast Diet fan. She says 'There is no need for your Fast Day meals to be punishing. This punchy puttanesca is low-fat and low-calorie but incredibly satisfying. It only needs a salad to make it a meal.' Romaine lettuce would be a good choice.

Serves six

1 tbsp extra virgin olive oil
20 anchovy fillets (drained); use fewer if you prefer a milder flavour
4 garlic cloves, peeled and roughly chopped
600g cherry tomatoes (orange 'Sungold' will give extra sweetness)
3 tbsps good-quality, mixed marinated olives (stoned)
2 tbsps capers (if salted, rinse before using)
12 boned, skinned chicken thighs
bunch of fresh basil (approximately 30g), stems removed
salt and pepper

Preheat oven to 180°C/350°F. Heat the olive oil in a heavy-based casserole dish (shallow works best). Add anchovies and garlic and gently fry for 2-3 minutes, until the anchovies have melted, but the garlic has not browned. Add cherry tomatoes, olives and capers, and turn down heat to simmer gently for 5 minutes. Then add the chicken thighs to the tomato mixture and stir well to combine. Place a lid on the casserole and position on a middle shelf in the oven. Cook for 15 minutes, then remove from the oven, give the chicken a good stir so it's well coated in the puttanesca sauce. Put back into the oven without the lid and cook for a further 20 minutes. Remove and allow to cool for a few minutes, before stirring in the basil leaves. Check for seasoning and serve.

NB

CHERRY TOMATOES CONTAIN LYCOPENE, AN ANTIOXIDANT THAT HELPS THE BODY FIGHT DISEASE

LO-LO MEATBALLS WITH CAVOLO NERO

CALORIE COUNT: **264**

Lo-lo, because much of the saturated fat you'd usually find in a typical Italian mamma meatball has been stripped out by swapping to a leaner meat and eliminating all but the merest flash of oil. And cavolo nero? Because it just sounds so great, the musketeer of the veg world. Besides, cavolo nero – a cultivar of kale – is tasty, nutritious, easy to grow and, yes, somehow *glamorous*.

Serves two

For the meatballs:
200g lean pork mince
  (or turkey mince)
½ medium red onion, chopped
1 garlic clove, peeled and crushed
1 small carrot, grated
pinch of oregano
1 egg, beaten
salt and pepper
oil for spraying

For the tomato sauce:
oil for spraying
½ medium red onion, chopped
½ garlic clove, peeled and chopped
1 400g tin chopped tomatoes
50g fresh tomatoes, skinned
  and deseeded, roughly chopped
1 tsp tomato purée
pinch of sugar
200ml water
chilli flakes to taste
dash of Worcestershire sauce
1 tsp dried oregano

For the cavolo nero:
200g cavolo nero, steamed
squeeze of lemon
sea salt

Place mince in a bowl with onion, garlic, carrot, oregano, egg and salt and pepper. Mix well and shape into 12 small meatballs. Spray a large pan with oil and fry over a medium heat until gently browned – about 4 minutes – and set aside. For the sauce, spray the same pan with oil and fry onion until softened; add garlic, and cook for a further 3 minutes. Add the tomatoes, tinned and fresh, purée, sugar and water, plus chilli flakes and Worcestershire sauce to taste. Simmer till reduced and glossy. Add meatballs and oregano, cover and simmer for 20 minutes. Serve with plenty of steamed cavolo, dressed with a light squeeze of lemon and a scatter of flaked sea salt.

NB

PORK CONTAINS ZINC NEEDED FOR A HEALTHY IMMUNE SYSTEM, AND THIS DISH PROVIDES A THIRD OF YOUR RDA

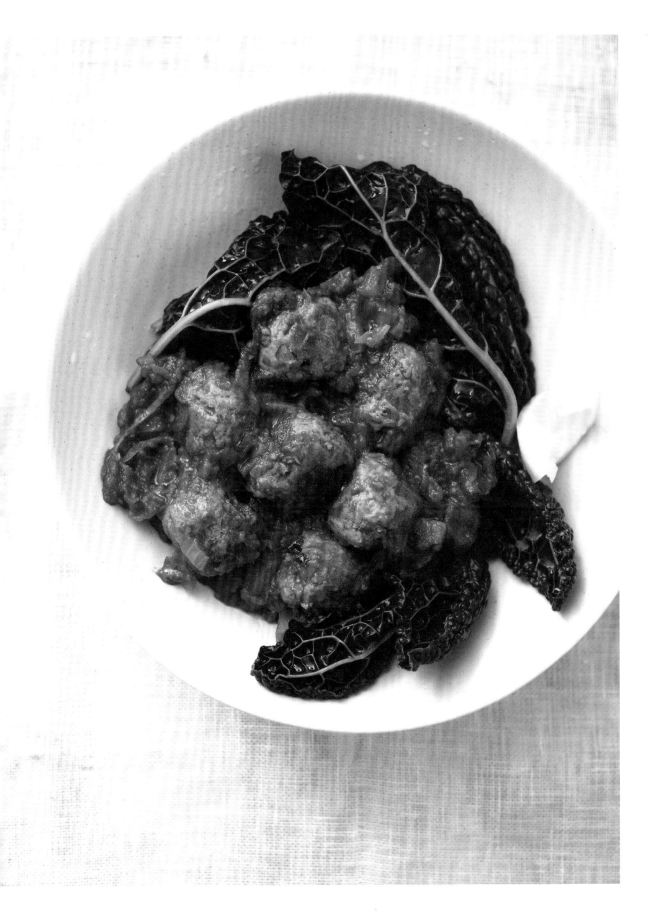

SARAH RAVEN'S PAN-FRIED LAMBS' KIDNEYS WITH LENTILS

CALORIE COUNT: **269**

For those who love kidneys this is hard to beat. Be careful not to overcook them: to be at their most tender the kidneys should be just turning from pink to brown, which takes less than 5 minutes.

Serves six

For the lentils:
300g Puy lentils
500ml vegetable or chicken stock
1 400g tin chopped tomatoes
1 tbsp extra virgin olive oil
2 garlic cloves, peeled and whole
1 head celery, finely sliced
1 fennel bulb, finely sliced
2 carrots, sliced
2 red chillies, seeds left in, chopped

3 bay leaves
large sprig of thyme

For the kidneys:
1 tbsp olive oil
14 lamb's kidneys (about 500g),
  halved and deveined
salt and pepper
large bunch of flat-leaf parsley,
  finely chopped

Put the lentils into a saucepan with the stock. Add the tomatoes, oil, whole garlic cloves, vegetables, chillies, bay leaves and thyme and cook gently for about 20 minutes, until the lentils begin to soften but not collapse. Add a little more stock or water if necessary to prevent them from boiling dry.

Heat the oil in a large frying pan and quickly fry the kidneys until just cooked. Stir in the lentils. Take the pan off the heat, season and add plenty of finely chopped parsley before serving.

NB

KIDNEYS CONTAIN HALF THE FAT OF LEAN RED MEAT, YET DOUBLE THE IRON AND 20 TIMES THE SELENIUM

LEMON-SCENTED STICKY CHICKEN WITH ROASTED VEGGIES

CALORIE COUNT: 287

The kids adore this – and it makes a light alternative to a traditional roast with all the big-boy trimmings. The idea is to fling everything in a pan and go away while the heat works its magic on the sweet lemon, and the chicken settles down to bless the veg with juice and flavour (a really good chicken is imperative). Just keep an eye that the veg at the edge isn't blackening too much. Otherwise, it's simply a case of feet up, crossword out. You may, of course, miss the roast potatoes. No matter. Cook them another day.

Serves four

1 medium free-range chicken
2 lemons (1 to place in the cavity of the bird, the other to squeeze over)
1 tbsp olive oil
2 red onions, or 8 shallots
1 yellow pepper and 1 red pepper, deseeded and cut into chunks

2 vines of plum tomatoes
1 aubergine, roughly cubed
handful of fresh thyme
sprig of rosemary
salt and pepper

Preheat oven to 180°C/350°F. Place vegetables in a roasting pan, season and place chicken on top, rubbing oil into skin. Squeeze lemon juice over bird and veggies, and add husk to pan. Coarsely chop thyme leaves and sprinkle over skin, adding some to the interior of the chicken together with the rosemary. Cook for an hour or more, until juices run clear. Halfway through cooking, check that the vegetables are not burning around the edges and move them around in the pan, tucking them under the chicken if necessary. Remove chicken from oven and allow to rest for 5 minutes, allowing the veggies cool slightly (room temperature is fine). Carve and serve on a generous mound of the sticky, lemony char-roasted veggies.

NB

PEPPERS ARE A GREAT SOURCE OF VITAMIN C, VITAL IN THE MANUFACTURE OF COLLAGEN, AN IMPORTANT STRUCTURAL PROTEIN

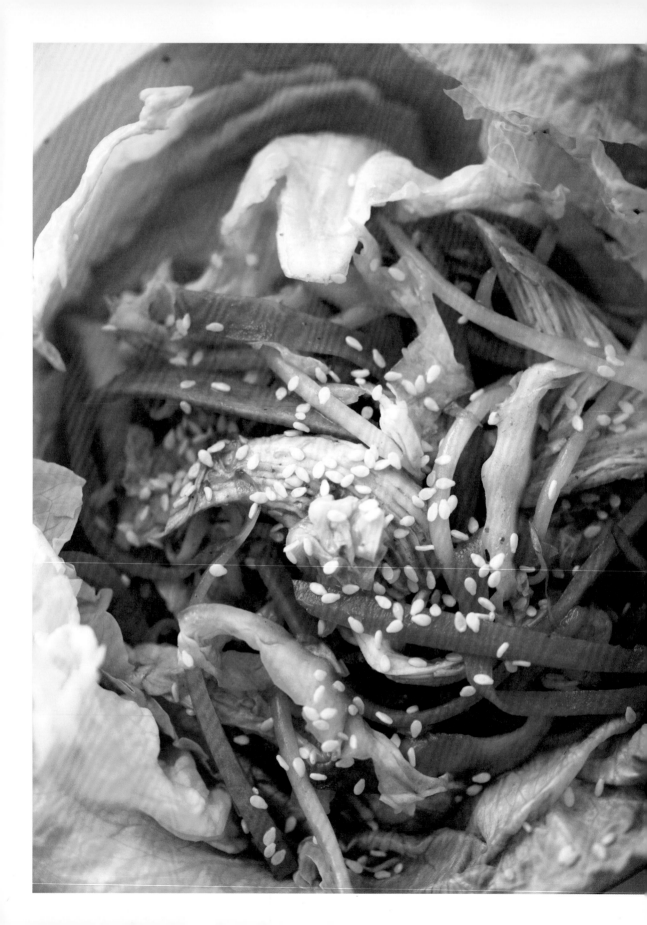

LETTUCE BOWLS WITH SHIITAKE AND HOISIN SHREDDED CHICKEN

CALORIE COUNT: **329**

A Fast Day version of a Chinese standard, and perhaps one for a day when you're feeling frilly and creative. You could add a little chopped water chestnut for extra crunch – they're only a calorie a gram.

oil for spraying
1 tsp root ginger, grated
1 tsp garlic, crushed
¼ Chinese cabbage, shredded
1 carrot, julienned
50g oyster mushrooms, chopped
50g shiitake mushrooms, chopped
50g beansprouts
ground white pepper
1 tbsp hoisin sauce
1 cooked chicken breast, shredded
2-3 iceberg lettuce leaves
½ tsp toasted sesame seeds

Heat a wok and spray with oil. Add ginger and garlic and stir-fry for 30 seconds. Add cabbage, carrot, mushrooms and beansprouts. Fry for 2-3 minutes until vegetables are just cooked but retain their bite. Season with pepper and add hoisin sauce. Add shredded chicken and toss to mix. Place 2 or 3 iceberg lettuce leaves in a wide-rimmed cup, making a bowl effect. Spoon chicken mixture into the bowl and serve with a scatter of toasted sesame seeds.

NB

EXOTIC MUSHROOMS CONTAIN ANTIOXIDANTS THAT GUARD AGAINST CELL DAMAGE AND HELP PREVENT TUMOUR GROWTH[24]

WARMING WINTER STEW

CALORIE COUNT: **385**

Fast Day food needn't be all about leaves and lemongrass. Here, I've taken a great British classic and modified it to bump up the veg and shout down the calories. On a non-Fast Day, you might have it with mash. But, really, it's a meal in itself without.

Serves four

1 tsp olive oil
1 onion, diced
handful of fresh sage leaves
400g good stewing steak or beef skirt,
   cut into chunks, fat removed
salt and pepper
2 tsps plain flour
2 parsnips, peeled and quartered
4 carrots, peeled and halved
½ small butternut squash, deseeded and
   roughly chopped (no need to peel)
3 Jerusalem artichokes, peeled and halved
2 tbsps tomato purée
1 bay leaf
250ml red wine
285ml vegetable stock
zest of a lemon, finely grated
rosemary leaves

Preheat oven to 170°C/325°F. Put oil in a casserole pan, add onion and sage leaves and fry for 3 minutes. Dust meat with seasoned flour and add to pan with the vegetables, tomato purée, bay leaf, wine and stock. Stir gently and season. Bring to the boil, cover with a lid, and cook in oven until the meat is tender and falls apart easily – about 3 hours. Garnish with lemon zest and a scatter of rosemary leaves.

NB

THE VEGGIES IN THIS STEW ARE LOW GI SO WILL HELP REGULATE APPETITE

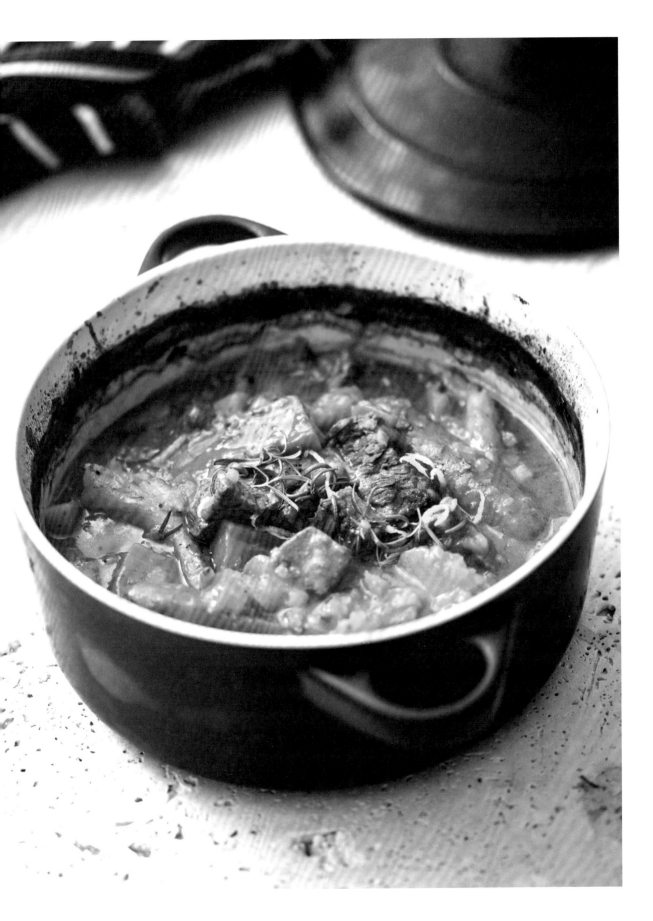

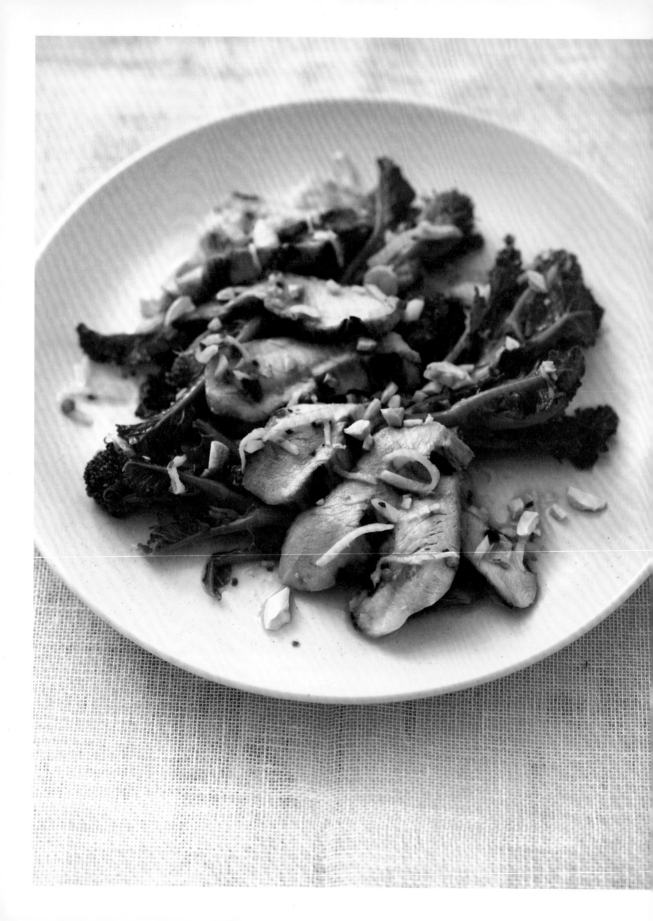

THE GINGER MAN'S GRIDDLED PHEASANT

CALORIE COUNT: **416**

In my home town of Brighton, only one man really rules the restaurant roost – The Ginger Man. Ben McKellar is a local fixture and we'd be lost without him. So here's his take on a pheasant salad, modified for us Fasters. It's the first time, incidentally, that The Ginger Man has ever concerned himself with calories when writing a recipe…

1 tsp root ginger, finely chopped
2 tbsps Thai fish sauce
pinch of chilli flakes
1 clove garlic, peeled and chopped
1 tsp raw agave nectar
juice of a lime
2 tbsps water
a few coriander leaves, chopped
1 skinless pheasant breast
100g broccoli florets
1 tsp chopped peanuts to serve

Mix the ginger, fish sauce, chilli flakes, garlic, agave, lime juice, water and coriander to make a chilli sauce. Marinate the pheasant breast in half of this mixture and set aside for up to 6 hours. Steam the broccoli for 6 minutes and keep warm. Cook the seasoned pheasant breast in a hot griddle pan until done to your liking, perhaps 4 minutes on each side. Slice the pheasant thinly, arrange on a plate with the broccoli and drizzle with the rest of the sauce. Add the chopped peanuts and serve.

NB

PHEASANT IS JUST AS RICH IN IRON AS BEEF

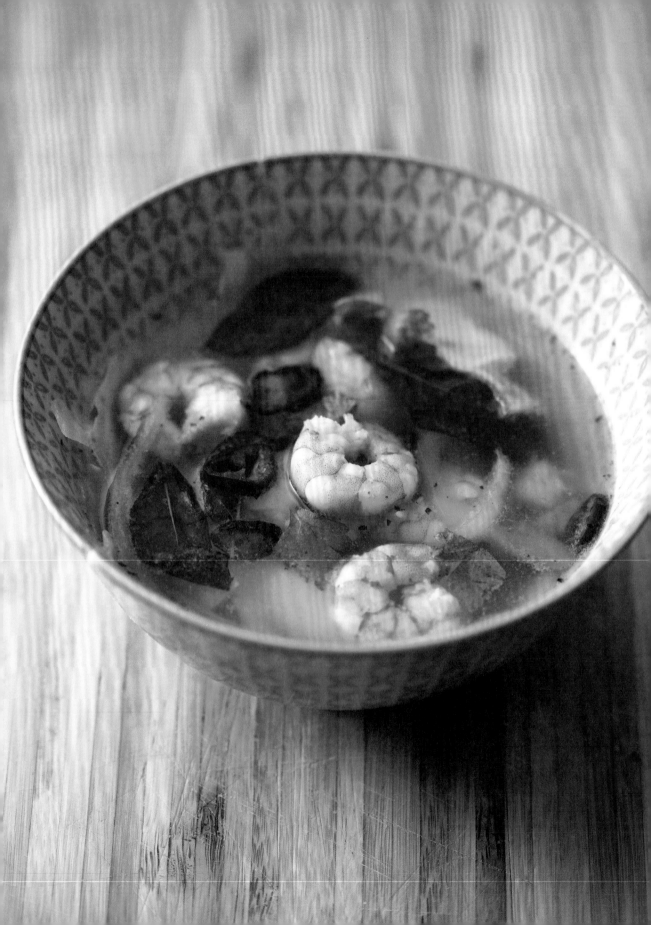

soups

FRAGRANT PHO

CALORIE COUNT: **48** ADD 15 FOR 50G EXTRA VEG

When travelling in Laos and Vietnam a decade ago, I came to adore the fresh, vivid taste of pho, served at every truck stop and roadside stall. This is a deliberately loose recipe – add spring vegetables of your choosing, anything that's going spare in the salad drawer, the veg box, the windowsill herb pot or the allotment. The quality of taste hinges on a good stock, so do contemplate making your own.

Serves four

2 lemongrass stems, outer leaves
  removed, inner stem finely chopped
2 tsps grated root ginger
4 kaffir lime leaves, torn
1500ml vegetable or fish stock
1 tsp palm sugar

3 tbsps Thai fish sauce
juice of a lime
8 large prawns, shelled and deveined
fresh Thai basil leaves, mint, coriander
  and finely sliced red chilli to serve

Use a pestle and mortar to grind lemongrass, ginger and kaffir lime leaves. Add to a large saucepan with stock and boil for 10 minutes. Add palm sugar, fish sauce and lime juice, tasting to check for balance. Cook prawns in the broth till pink – about 2-3 minutes. Add herbs and red chilli to serve.

To bulk up the broth, add mangetouts, sugar snap peas, shredded spring cabbage, ribboned carrots, beansprouts, shiitake mushrooms or baby sweetcorn along with the prawns.

NB

STUDIES SHOW THAT SOUP INCREASES SATIATION – AND STOPS YOU OVER-EATING[25]

CLEAR TOFU BROTH

CALORIE COUNT: **54**

Plenty of us crave clean, clear flavour on a Fast Day, and this tofu broth fits the bill. There's something vibrant and sparky about its combination of ginger, spring onion and coriander. You somehow know instinctively that it is a Good Thing.

Serves four

1200ml clear vegetable stock
100g baby sweetcorn
1 tsp root ginger, julienned
3 spring onions, finely chopped
3 tsps soy sauce
2 tsps mirin
1 tsp rice wine vinegar
225g tofu, diced
50g beansprouts
coriander leaves to garnish

Heat stock till boiling, then add sweetcorn, ginger and spring onion. Simmer for 3-5 minutes, then add soy, mirin, vinegar, tofu and beansprouts. Season, simmer for a further minute and serve garnished with coriander leaves.

NB

REGULAR CONSUMPTION OF GINGER MAY HELP REDUCE BODY WEIGHT[26]

ROAST RED PEPPER SOUP

CALORIE COUNT: 58

Roasting with a drizzle of olive oil will bring sweetness and intensity to peppers and tomatoes, at the limited cost of a few additional calories. You could cover them for 10 minutes after roasting and then remove their peel for a silkier soup.

Serves four

3 large red peppers
3 ripe plum tomatoes, halved
1 onion, quartered
3 garlic cloves, peeled
1 tbsp olive oil
salt and pepper
pinch of caster sugar
1 tsp cumin seeds
chilli flakes to taste
juice and husk of half a lemon
1200ml chicken stock
2 tsps tomato purée
1 tsp balsamic vinegar
basil leaves to serve

Preheat oven to 200°C/400°F. Place peppers, tomatoes, onion and garlic in a roasting pan. Drizzle with oil, season, add sugar, cumin seeds, chilli flakes and lemon juice, plus husk, and roast until slightly caramelised – around 20 minutes. Transfer to a large saucepan, remove lemon husk, and add stock and tomato purée. Bring to boil and simmer for 10 minutes, removing any floating tomato skins. Transfer to a processor, or use a hand-blender, re-season, add the vinegar and purée until smooth. Add more stock if necessary to achieve desired consistency. Serve garnished with basil leaves.

NB

ROASTING THE PEPPERS HELPS RELEASE THE CAROTENOIDS; THE ADDITION OF OIL IMPROVES THEIR ABSORPTION INTO THE BODY

BLOODY MARY SOUP

CALORIE COUNT: 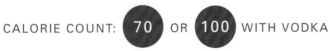 OR 100 WITH VODKA

This is rocks-off tomato soup – packed with spiky flavour and (if you want) a jolt of vodka. It is served hot, with the usual Bloody Mary accompaniments of lemon, celery, Tabasco and Lea & Perrins. Ditch the vodka, of course, to cut back on Fast Day calories.

Serves four

1kg ripe tomatoes, skinned and halved
2 red chillies, halved and deseeded
salt and pepper
½ tsp caster sugar
1½ tsps olive oil
1 litre vegetable stock
1 tbsp tomato purée
1 tsp horseradish sauce
1 tbsp Worcestershire sauce
1 tbsp dry sherry
4 tbsps vodka (optional)
4 celery stalks, and leaves
Tabasco, cracked black pepper, celery
    salt and lemon slices to serve

Preheat oven to 200°C/400°F. Place tomato halves and chillies, sprinkled with seasoning and sugar, in a roasting pan. Drizzle with oil and bake till softened, about 20 minutes. Purée in a blender, adding a little stock to loosen. Transfer to a saucepan, adding remaining stock and tomato purée. Heat through without boiling. Add horseradish, Worcestershire sauce, sherry and vodka (if using). Check seasoning and serve in thick glasses, with Tabasco, cracked black pepper, celery salt, celery stalks and lemon slices. This also works as a cold soup.

NB

CELERY IS SAID TO HAVE 'NEGATIVE CALORIES': ONE STICK CONTAINS ABOUT 2 CALORIES, BUT THE ENERGY COST OF EATING AND DIGESTING IT FAR OUTWEIGHS THIS

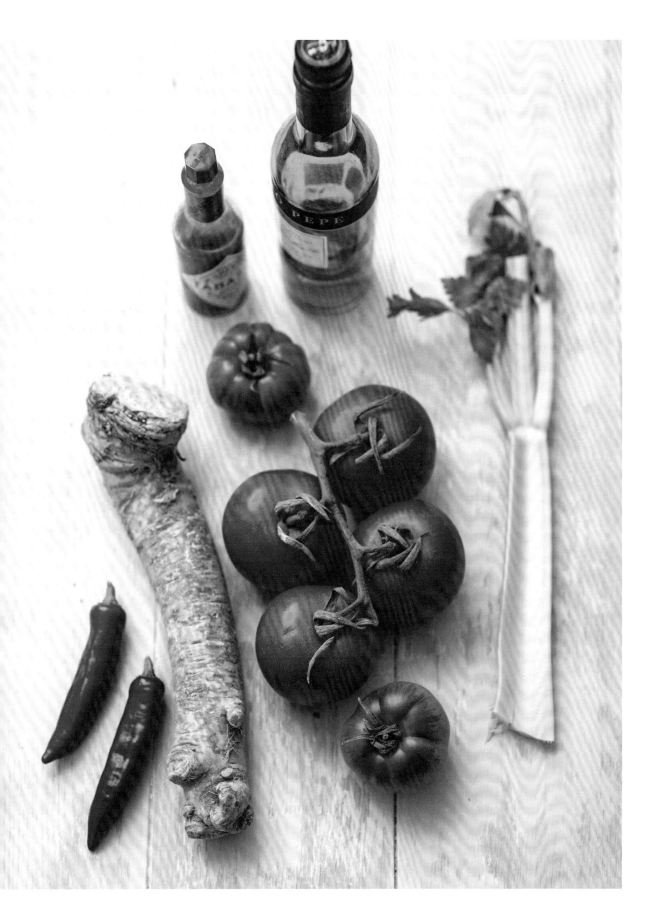

SOMERSET NETTLE SOUP

CALORIE COUNT: **77** OR **126** WITH HALF-FAT CRÈME FRAÎCHE

There's something about soup recipes that makes them wonderfully communal – something to share among friends. This one is from my mate Marcus, who lives near Wincanton and is rarely away from his beloved Aga and its bubbling stockpots. It's a soup for believers: you need to be a forager, and you need a pair of sturdy gloves. Says Marcus, 'This soup works best in the spring when the nettles are young. Older nettles become slightly woody and can give a bitter taste to the soup. Pick just the tops of the nettles – the leaves lower down are tougher and hairier, while the stems will be thicker.' He also advises going big: 'If you're foraging, you might as well do it in bulk. The soup will freeze well enough.'

Serves 10-12

a carrier bag full of young nettle tops
1 tbsp rapeseed oil
3 large onions, sliced
3 celery stalks, chopped
2 carrots, chopped
4 garlic cloves – or 2 large handfuls of wild garlic leaves, if available
4 litres chicken or veg stock
good grating of nutmeg
salt and pepper
low-fat crème fraîche and snipped chives or parsley to serve

Wash the nettles and remove any non-nettle foliage, any bugs and the thicker stems. Heat the oil in a large tall-sided pan and sweat the onions, celery, carrots and garlic (but not the wild garlic leaves, if using), until softened. Add the stock and nettles (and wild garlic leaves). Bring to the boil and simmer until the nettle leaves are tender, up to 10 minutes. Liquidise the soup in a processor, or use a hand-held blender, then season and add nutmeg to taste. Serve with a spoonful of crème fraîche, snipped chives or parsley – or more of the wild garlic leaves.

NB

NETTLES CONTAIN COMPOUNDS THAT CAN IMPROVE HEALTH AND PREVENT CANCER[27]

RED VELVET SOUP

CALORIE COUNT: **87** OR **107** WITH BREADSTICK

A dense crimson broth for those soupy days when you want to do little more than curl up on the sofa and cuddle the cat.

Serves four

1 tbsp olive oil
1 onion, finely chopped
1 garlic clove, peeled and crushed
a pinch of caster sugar
1 tbsp tomato purée
1kg ripe red tomatoes, skinned and roughly chopped
1 bay leaf
fresh thyme
600ml water
salt and pepper

Heat oil in a large pan and sauté onions until softened but not browned. Add garlic, sugar, tomato purée and tomatoes. Add bay and thyme, tied together for easy removal, and the water. Bring to boil, then reduce to a simmer for 15-20 minutes. Remove herbs and blend soup until smooth and velvety. Check consistency, adding a little hot water if necessary. Reheat, season and serve with a grissini breadstick.

NB

TOMATOES CONTAIN SUBSTANCES THAT GUARD AGAINST CANCER, BUT RESEARCH SUGGESTS THEY MAY ALSO HELP PREVENT NEURODEGENERATIVE DISEASES SUCH AS ALZHEIMER'S[28]

SUMMERTIME SPECIAL SOUP

CALORIE COUNT: **91**

Cooking with lettuce may not promise many thrills, but here its fresh green clarity
– teamed with that of the cucumber and trumped by the glory of fresh shelled
peas – works wonders. Frozen peas are fine. This cold soup is just the thing to
eat as spring gets underway and the evenings start to lengthen.

Serves four

1 tsp vegetable oil
4 spring onions, chopped
1 round lettuce, shredded
1 large cucumber, peeled, deseeded
  and roughly chopped
150g fresh or frozen peas
1 litre vegetable stock
1 vegetable stock cube
salt and pepper
snipped chives
1 tbsp half-fat crème fraîche

Heat oil in a large pan and add spring onions, cooking gently for 3 minutes. Add
lettuce, cucumber and peas, stir and sweat for 5 minutes. Add stock and stock
cube, season and bring to the boil. Reduce heat and simmer with lid on for 15
minutes. Cool and blitz with a hand-held blender. Refrigerate until cold, check
seasoning and consistency, and serve with chives and a swirl of crème fraîche.

NB

FROZEN PEAS OFTEN CONTAIN MORE VITAMIN C THAN WEEK-OLD FRESH PEAS; FREEZING JUST
AFTER PICKING LOCKS IN THE VITAMIN WHICH OTHERWISE DECLINES OVER TIME

CARROT AND GINGER

CALORIE COUNT: 93

Very low in calories, very pretty, very been-there-done-that – until you bring in star anise, cinnamon, cumin and ginger. Then? *Ka-pow.*

Serves two

1 tsp sunflower oil
1 onion, diced
1 star anise
1 tsp root ginger, grated
100g carrots, grated
½ cinnamon stick
600ml vegetable stock
cumin seeds and coriander to serve

Sweat the onion in a pan with oil, star anise and ginger. Add carrots, cinnamon stick and stock, and simmer for 15-20 minutes. Remove star anise and cinnamon, blend and serve with a scatter of cumin seeds and fresh coriander leaves.

NB

THERE IS GROWING EVIDENCE THAT CINNAMON HELPS CONTROL BLOOD SUGAR LEVELS[29]

ARAB SPRING VEGETABLE BROTH

CALORIE COUNT: 102

This delicious, clear soup is inspired by *Moro*, one of the most thumbed (and sauce-stained) cookbooks on my kitchen shelf. Chefs Sam and Sam Clark have long used the flavours of Iberia and North Africa to great effect; the point here is a simple melody of taste, transferred from morning market to piping hot soup bowl without much to-do. I've added sumac for a lemony kick.

Serves four

1250ml chicken stock – home-made will give the best flavour
   to such an elegant soup
150g broad beans, podded
150g peas, fresh or frozen
6 asparagus spears, cut into 2cm pieces, woody stems removed
2 globe artichokes, trimmed, quartered and very finely sliced
generous handful of fresh mint, flat-leaf parsley and coriander, chopped
2 spring onions, finely chopped
1 tbsp sumac
juice of half a lemon
salt and pepper
4 thin rye crispbreads to serve

Heat stock in a large pan, bring to a gentle simmer and add vegetables. Cook for 2 minutes until tender. Remove pan from heat and add herbs, spring onion, sumac and lemon juice. Season carefully (sumac can be salty). Serve in white bowls with shards of broken crispbread.

NB

THIS SOUP PROVIDES RESPECTABLE AMOUNTS OF POTASSIUM, MAGNESIUM, IRON AND ZINC, AS WELL AS THE VITAMINS FOLATE, NIACIN, A AND C

SPINACH, SORREL AND NUTMEG

CALORIE COUNT: **102** OR **185** WITH A POACHED EGG

Now we're talking: a glorious, nutritious bowl of jolly green goodness which is, if such a thing were possible, the Fast Diet distilled into a single spoonful. Try to find sorrel if you can (it's easy to grow) – it lends an acidic tang here and is well worth the search. If you have spare calories floating around, pop a poached egg on top and marvel at your delightful bowl of good green gold.

Serves four

1 tbsp olive oil
1 medium onion, diced
1 garlic clove, peeled and crushed
1250ml chicken or vegetable stock
½ tsp root ginger, chopped
grating of nutmeg to taste
salt and pepper
500g spinach leaves, washed
125g sorrel leaves
2 tbsps low-fat crème fraîche
thyme leaves to serve

Heat oil in a large saucepan and sauté onion and garlic until softened but not coloured. Add stock, ginger and nutmeg and bring to the boil. Season and simmer for 10 minutes. Add spinach and sorrel (dandelion leaves work well too), and cook for a further 2 minutes. Remove from heat and stir in crème fraîche. Adjust seasoning, check consistency and serve with picked thyme leaves.

NB

NUTMEG CONTAINS A SUBSTANCE CALLED MACELIGNAN WHICH CAN HELP PROTECT TEETH AGAINST CARIES[30]

ALLOTMENT SOUP

CALORIE COUNT: 108

This is a glut in a bowl and, as such, defies rules. My only suggestion would be to try it semi-smooth – half of it fully blitzed, the other left chunky, then recombined prior to serving. It makes for an engaging texture, and promises to fill you up as soon as you look at it. The smoked paprika, too, adds a cunning twist.

Serves four

1 tbsp olive oil
500g non-starchy vegetables of your
   choice: courgettes, spinach, peppers, kale,
   cavolo nero, leeks – whatever you have a
   glut of, or whatever is cheap and plentiful in
   the shops
400g tomatoes, skinned and roughly
   chopped
1 large onion, chopped
2 carrots, peeled and chopped

2 celery stalks, chopped
2 garlic cloves, peeled and crushed
1 tsp smoked paprika
1500ml vegetable stock, made from veg
   trimmings boiled for 20 minutes
   with bouquet garni, then strained
garden herbs of choice – perhaps chervil,
   marjoram, thyme
salt and pepper

Heat oil in a large pan, add chopped vegetables, garlic and smoked paprika, and sweat for 5 minutes. Add stock, season and allow to simmer gently for 20 minutes. Cool slightly, then blitz half of the soup in a food processor, or with a hand-held blender, keeping the remaining half as it is. Return blitzed half to pan with the non-blitzed half and reheat, stirring to achieve a semi-smooth soup. Serve topped with a tangle of herbs from the garden.

NB

THE ONLY NUTRIENT MISSING FROM THIS SOUP IS VITAMIN B12 (AND THAT'S BECAUSE IT'S ONLY FOUND IN ANIMAL PROTEINS)

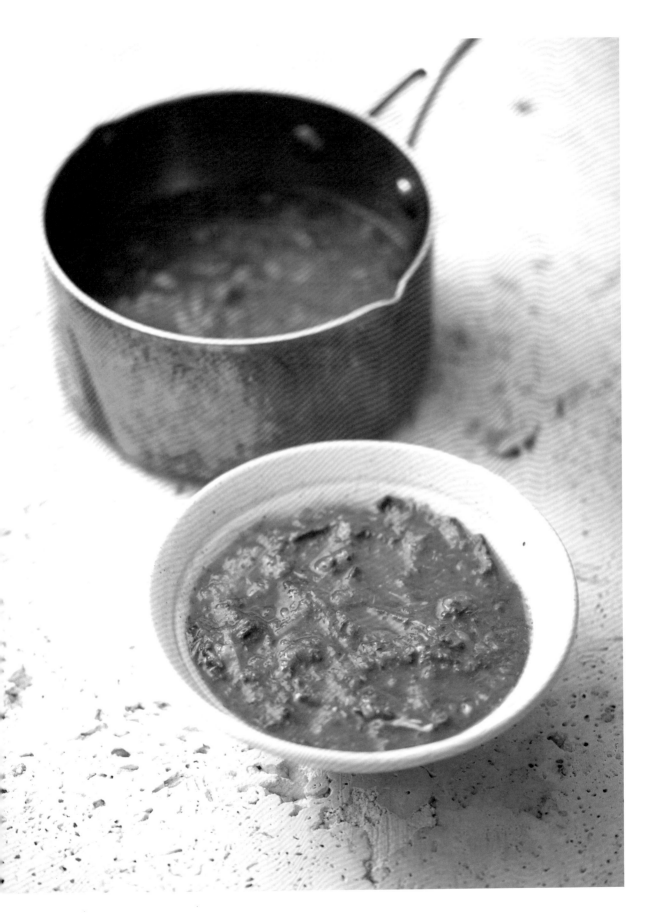

GAZPACHO THREE WAYS

Classic Spanish

CALORIE COUNT: 113

This is about as simple as soup can be – the very essence of summer, served fridge-cold and packed with wonderful flavour and impeccable nutritional cred. This recipe is a classic version, given to me by my Pilates teacher Ana, who grew up in Spain. The original recipe dates from Roman times and contained bread. You don't need it.

Serves two

1 red pepper, deseeded and coarsely chopped
300g red tomatoes, ideally a mix of varieties
½ cucumber (150-200g), chopped

1 red chilli, deseeded and chopped
1 garlic clove, peeled
2 spring onions, sliced
2 tbsps red wine vinegar
1 tbsp good olive oil
6 ice cubes (if you're in a hurry)
salt and pepper

To garnish:
Finely diced cucumber, tomato and spring onion

Purée the raw vegetables, including the chilli, garlic and spring onion, in a food processor until smooth. Add vinegar, olive oil, salt and pepper and quickly blitz again. Serve cold with garnish. Gazpacho does not freeze well, so serve fresh.

Fiery roasted gazpacho

CALORIE COUNT: 113

First oven-roast the tomatoes, peppers and chilli, sprinkled with 2 tsps paprika. Allow to cool and blend with other the ingredients as above.

To make a heartier meal and include protein, serve with: a sprinkle of crab meat (50g, add 40 cals) and lemon zest; or a crumble of feta (30g, add 100 cals); or with a chopped hard-boiled egg (add 60 cals) and a pinch of salt.

Green gazpacho

CALORIE COUNT: 277

A cool alternative to traditional gazpacho, especially if you're not overly fond of tomatoes.

Serves two

1 celery stalk (including leaves), roughly chopped
1 small green pepper, deseeded and roughly chopped
½ cucumber, peeled and chopped
½ avocado, chopped
1 green chilli (or less, to taste), chopped
1 tsp Tabasco
2 garlic cloves, peeled
½ tsp sugar
100g baby spinach

30g walnuts
handful of basil leaves
handful of curly parsley
2 tbsps sherry vinegar
1 tbsp olive oil
1 tbsp low-fat natural yoghurt
250ml water
4 ice cubes
salt and pepper

Blitz all ingredients in a food processor, including the ice cubes. Add water in stages to achieve desired consistency. Season and serve.

NB

CAPSAICIN, THE ACTIVE INGREDIENT IN CHILLI, HAS BEEN SHOWN TO INCREASE ENERGY EXPENDITURE AND IMPROVE SATIETY[31]

BEETROOT AND BRAMLEY SOUP WITH HORSERADISH

CALORIE COUNT: 116

The idea for this tangy autumn soup came from my friend Alex Renton, who made it for me one chilly lunchtime at his home in Edinburgh. I loved it so much that I made it for chef Allegra McEvedy, who asked to use it in her *Guardian* column, and now it's turning up here, a triumph of recipe recycling. This is the Fast Day version – no butter for sweating the onion, a swirl of yoghurt instead of cream – but it's no less tasty than the original. It freezes like a dream, so you could double the quantities and have it handy as the nights draw in.

Serves four

500g raw beetroot
2 medium onions, roughly chopped
1 tbsp olive oil
2 Bramley apples, peeled, quartered
   and cored with a squeeze of lemon
   to prevent discolouration

1½ litres light chicken
   or vegetable stock
2 star anise
snipped chives
salt and pepper
1 tsp horseradish sauce
1 tbsp natural low-fat yoghurt

Preheat the oven to 200°C/400°F. Place the beetroot in 1cm water in a baking tray. Cook for an hour, or until a knife meets with little resistance, then take them out and run under cold water for a couple of minutes until cool enough to peel.

Heat the oil in a thick-bottomed pan. Add onions and sweat over a medium heat with the lid on until soft but not coloured. Add apple quarters. Roughly chop the peeled beetroots and add to the pan. Pour on the stock, add star anise and seasoning and simmer for 15 minutes. Remove star anise, then blitz the soup with a hand blender until puréed. Serve with snipped chives and a swirl of yoghurt mixed with the horseradish sauce.

NB

BEETROOT CONTAINS DIETARY NITRATE, WHICH MAY HELP TO IMPROVE EXERCISE PERFORMANCE [32]

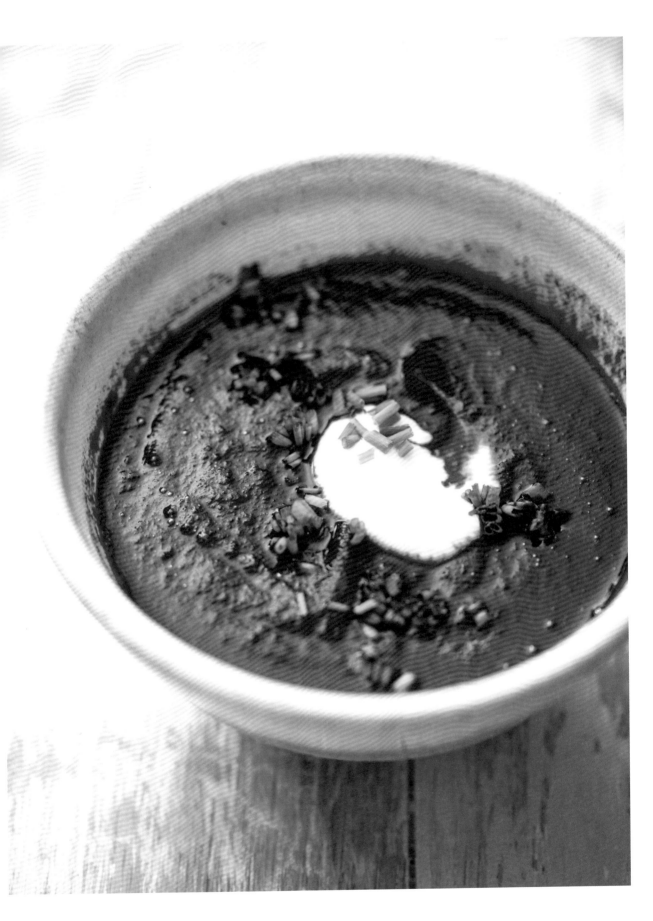

SHIITAKE NOODLE DASHI

CALORIE COUNT: **137**

This soup starts with a simple dashi – a Japanese stock that can be used as a base for countless soups. In Japan, sea vegetables are the heart of many dishes, but they're something we tend to ignore in the West – which is a shame, as seaweed, in all its many forms, is high in minerals, including iodine, potassium, calcium and iron. And it's low in calories, of course. Dashi-kombu is sun-dried and cut into various sizes, then soaked to unlock the kelp's unique unami flavour. Rinse it first to wash away the salt of the drying process.

To make the dashi stock:
750ml water
3 slices kombu seaweed, approximately 10cm long
5 dried shiitake mushrooms

Place kombu in water and slowly bring to a simmer (but do not boil) for about 10 minutes. Remove the kombu, add the dried mushrooms and boil for a further minute, then turn off the heat and allow to sit, uncovered, for 20 minutes. Remove the mushrooms and store the dashi for later use. It will keep for up to 5 days in the fridge, or freezes well.

For the soup:
350ml dashi stock
100g fresh shiitake mushrooms
100g rinsed shirataki noodles
1 tsp soy sauce
1 tsp mirin
½ tsp wasabi, or to taste
1 tsp root ginger, julienned
1 spring onion, finely chopped

Bring the dashi stock to a simmer in a pan and add the remaining soup ingredients. Heat through and add chopped spring onion to serve.

NB

KELP IS AN ASTONISHING PROVIDER OF CALCIUM – OVER A GRAM PER 100G

SKIPPER'S SOUP

CALORIE COUNT: **142**

A quick-fix, morale-boosting soup from food writer, seafarer and friend Alex Renton. This, he says, is smoky, spicy and full of fibre – great for cold days or after exercise, and easy to rustle up from store-cupboard ingredients, even in the galley below decks while a storm rages outside. It freezes well, so it makes sense to make a quantity and keep it in portion sizes. 'I always prefer home-made stock, though the calorie count will be higher than with a stock cube,' he adds. 'But if you sieve and chill the home-made stock after making it you can remove much of the fat.' Aye aye, skipper.

Serves one

25g good-quality chorizo
1 small onion, finely chopped
200g tinned haricot beans
   (cannellini, butter beans or chickpeas
   will work too), drained
300ml chicken stock
pinch of smoked paprika
salt and pepper

Chop the chorizo into small chunks and heat gently in a heavy-bottomed pan. When it has released some oil, add the onion and fry gently till softened. Add beans and stock and simmer for 10 minutes. Whizz with a hand blender until smooth. Add the paprika, check seasoning and serve, with a dollop of low-fat natural yoghurt if you can spare the calories (add 10 for a tbsp).

NB

THE FIBRE CONTENT HERE IS 7G PER PORTION, OVER A THIRD OF YOUR RDA

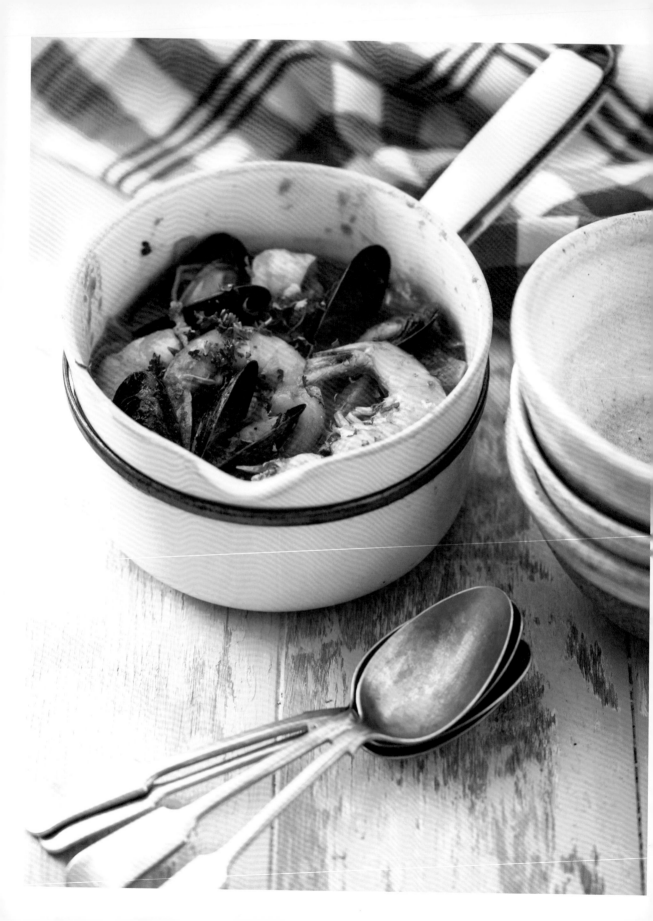

SKINNY BOUILLABAISSE

CALORIE COUNT: **163**

My sister Debs is a dab hand in the kitchen, having trained in the world-renowned kitchens at Ballymaloe in Ireland. This broth is designed to bring all the rounded, rich flavour of a traditional French fish stew to your low-calorie Fast Day soup bowl. Even without the usual butter, aioli and croûtes, this is still quite a flash dish. One to make when your Fast friends drop by. Notice the calorie count. Sing.

Serves four

1½ tsps olive oil
1 onion, finely sliced
1 fennel bulb, trimmed and finely sliced
4 garlic cloves, peeled and crushed
1 tsp root ginger, finely grated
1 red chilli, finely chopped (deseeded first, if you prefer less heat)
generous pinch of saffron threads
1 tsp paprika
1 400g tin chopped tomatoes

1250ml fish or vegetable stock
½ tsp caster sugar
1 bay leaf
400g white fish, cut into chunks
8 mussels, scrubbed
8 large raw king prawns, peeled and deveined, tails left on
salt and pepper
handful of flat-leaf parsley
lemon juice to taste

Heat olive oil in large heavy-based pan over medium heat; add onion and fennel and cook, stirring occasionally, for about 5 minutes until softened but not coloured. Add garlic, ginger, chilli, saffron and paprika and cook for a further 2 minutes until fragrant. Stir in tomatoes, stock, sugar and bay leaf, scraping pan with a wooden spoon to release any stickiness on the base. Season and simmer for 20-25 minutes. Gently lower the fish, mussels and prawns into the soup, cover the pan and cook for 2-3 minutes until fish and prawns are just opaque and mussels have opened (discarding any that have failed to open). Check the seasoning, scatter with parsley and add a squeeze of lemon juice to taste.

NB

ONLY 2G OF FAT, BUT A SUBSTANTIAL 28G OF PROTEIN PER SERVING – AND A TON OF TASTE

FAST DAY MINESTRONE

CALORIE COUNT: **228** OR **313** WITH PASTA

Minestrone means 'big soup' – and that's exactly what you'll get from this recipe. This is the heartland of Fast Diet cooking: filling but full of sunny flavour and packed with vital vits. The vegetables in a minestrone can, of course, vary according to your preference and what's in season. Try curly kale instead of spinach, asparagus instead of green beans, chickpeas or broad beans instead of cannellini, or throw in a handful of frozen peas towards the end of cooking. For speed and simplicity, you could simply add handfuls of frozen vegetables to your broth – peas, sweetcorn, carrots, broccoli. Sacrifice the pasta if you want to save on calories and GL. For minestrone verde, leave out the chopped tomatoes, stick to green veg and bump up the stock by 100ml.

Serves four

1 tbsp olive oil
1 onion, diced
1 clove garlic, peeled and chopped
3 celery stalks, chopped
1 small leek, diced
2 carrots, diced
1 litre vegetable or chicken stock
1 chicken stock cube
1 bay leaf

100g small pasta, perhaps orrechiette or conchigliette
1 400g tin chopped tomatoes
150g cannellini beans
100g French green beans, chopped
1 courgette, diced
100g baby spinach leaves
fresh oregano and basil leaves
salt and pepper
2 tsps Parmesan, grated, to serve

Heat the oil in a large pan and sauté onion and garlic until softened. Add celery, leek and carrots and cook this *soffritto* for a further 3-4 minutes until golden and flavourful. Add the stock, stock cube and bay leaf, and bring to the boil. Add pasta if using and cook for 4 minutes. Reduce heat and add chopped tomatoes, cannellini beans, green beans and courgette. Simmer for 2-4 minutes (depending on the cooking time of your chosen pasta), then add spinach leaves, herbs and seasoning. Serve with a little Parmesan and more fresh herbs.

NB

IF YOU WANT A LITTLE CARBOHYDRATE BUT FEWER CALORIES, SWAP THE PASTA FOR POTATO, WHICH WILL ONLY ADD 18

DEBS' CHICKEN NOODLE SOUP WITH AVOCADO AND CUCUMBER

CALORIE COUNT: **237**

This is my sister's take on the classic chicken noodle soup, beloved of Jewish mums and nursemaids everywhere. The addition of cucumber, avocado and lime makes for a novel spoonful. Truly a chicken noodle soup for the soul.

Serves four

100g rice noodles
1250ml home-made chicken stock
pinch of chilli flakes or finely chopped fresh
    chilli, to taste
2 skinless chicken breasts, thinly sliced
salt and pepper
pinch of caster sugar
½ iceberg lettuce, shredded
½ cucumber, diced
1 avocado, diced with a squeeze of lemon
    to prevent discolouration
2 spring onions, finely sliced
2 tbsps coriander leaves, roughly chopped
squeeze of lime

Cook noodles according to instructions, drain, refresh, drain again and set aside. Bring stock to the boil, add chilli flakes and chicken slices. Reduce heat, season, then add the sugar and simmer gently until chicken is cooked, about 4-5 minutes depending on size of chicken pieces. Divide lettuce, cucumber, avocado, spring onions and coriander between four hot soup bowls. Add noodles to hot broth, bring swiftly to the boil and pour over veggies. Add a squeeze of lime.

NB

AVOCADOS ARE A GREAT SOURCE OF ANTIOXIDANT VITAMIN E, IMPORTANT FOR THE IMMUNE SYSTEM

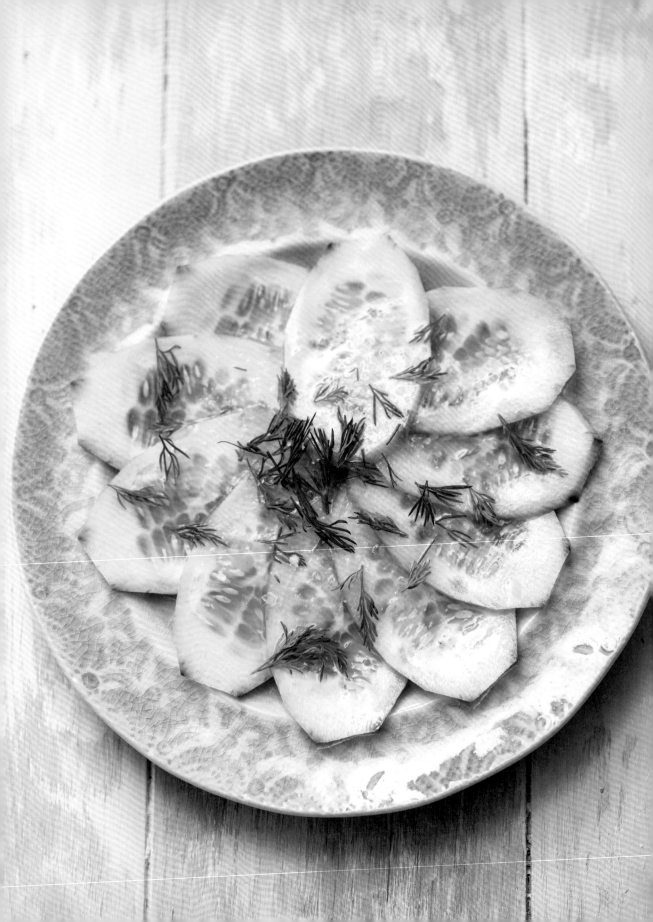

salads

SUMMER CUCUMBER SALAD WITH DILL

CALORIE COUNT: **43**

As simple a salad as was ever thrown together on a plate. It doesn't require fanfare. Just a fork.

Serves four as a side dish

1 large cucumber, peeled and thinly sliced

For the dressing:
1 tbsp mild olive oil
2 tsps Dijon mustard
2 tsps white wine vinegar
1 tsp caster sugar
salt and pepper
2 tbsps fresh dill, chopped

Place cucumber slices on a serving dish. Whisk dressing ingredients and add, finishing with a good grind of black pepper.

NB

IN A CLINICAL TRIAL, PATIENTS WITH METABOLIC SYNDROME GIVEN DILL FOR 12 WEEKS SHOWED A REDUCTION IN BLOOD LIPIDS[33]

FENNEL, CUCUMBER AND RADISH SALAD WITH A CITRUS VINAIGRETTE

CALORIE COUNT: **52**

A star of Italian cooking, fennel is only just finding its way into our hearts. It's a humble thing, but full of nutrients. According to researchers, the 'most fascinating phytonutrient compound in fennel' may be anethole – the primary component of its volatile oil. In animal studies, the anethole in fennel has repeatedly been shown to reduce inflammation and to help prevent the occurrence of cancer.[34] You needn't get too hung up on any of this, though. Just enjoy its sharp liquorice flavour, and don't grate your fingers on the mandolin.

Serves two

For the vinaigrette:
1 tsp lemongrass, finely chopped
1 tsp soy sauce
1 tsp sesame oil
3 tsps lime juice
pinch of sugar

For the salad:
1 fennel bulb, mandolined
½ cucumber, deseeded and sliced into
    thin crescents
200g assorted radishes (French
    breakfast, mooli, daikon), finely sliced
1 spring onion, finely chopped
½ tsp root ginger, grated
chilli flakes to taste
handful of young coriander and fresh
    mint leaves

Combine vinaigrette ingredients, assemble the salad and dress. Add a handful of chopped peanuts if your calorie budget allows (add 73 calories for 10).

NB

YOU'LL GET A QUARTER OF YOUR RDA OF POTASSIUM FROM THIS SALAD

ASPARAGUS SALAD WITH RED ONION AND GRIDDLED MUSHROOM

CALORIE COUNT: 110

Anyone who understands and adores seasonal cooking will know the thrill of the first asparagus arriving – as exciting as the Jersey Royals coming into season in April or the Victoria plums suddenly heavy on the trees. The British asparagus season traditionally begins on April 23 and ends on Midsummer's Day, which is delightfully specific – and I recommend you get stuck in (asparagus contains around 20 calories per 100g, as long as you don't treat it to a butter bath). Young asparagus may work best here, but don't overcook it. Treat it as you would vermouth in a martini and barely show it the heat. In, out, eat.

Serves four

1 tbsp olive oil
2 red onions, cut into eighths
4 large Portobello mushrooms, sliced
3 garlic cloves, peeled and crushed
3 courgettes, thickly sliced on the diagonal, blanched and refreshed
300g young asparagus, trimmed, briefly blanched and refreshed
salt and pepper
squeeze of lemon
2 tbsps Parmesan, grated or shaved, to serve

Heat oil in a large griddle pan and add onion, cook for 2 minutes and add sliced mushrooms. Griddle until softened and charred, turning often. Add garlic and courgette and continue to griddle for 3 more minutes. Place on a platter and top with a mess of asparagus, thrown on like pick-up-sticks. Season well, then add a squeeze of lemon and a generous sprinkling of Parmesan.

NB

THIS SUBSTANTIAL SALAD PROVIDES YOUR ENTIRE FOLATE REQUIREMENT FOR A DAY

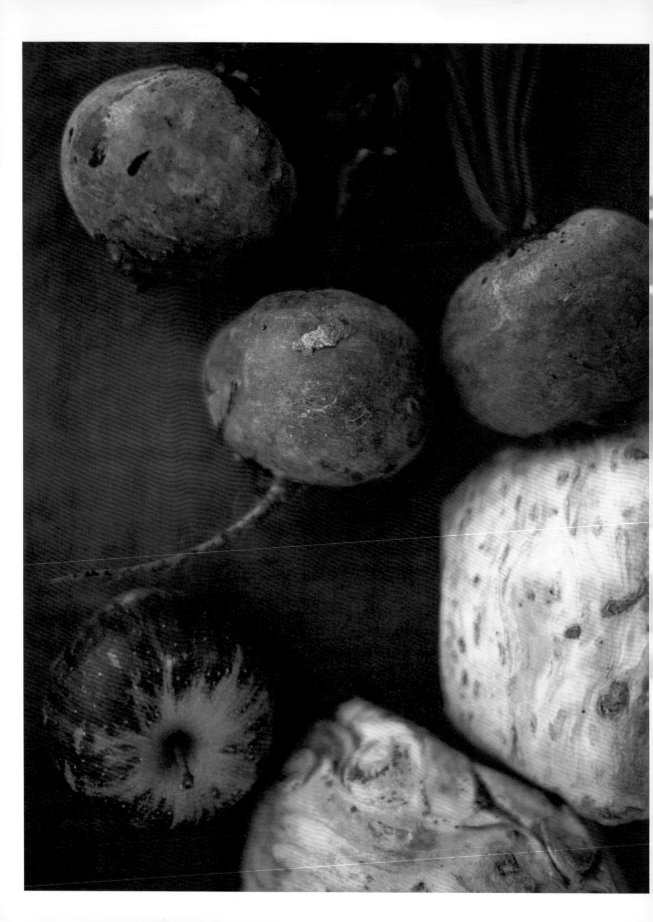

PENNY'S BEETROOT SALAD

CALORIE COUNT: 114

My dear friend Penny is a world-class beetroot queen, and this salad – a fiery mouthful of cumin, OJ, horseradish and mustard – is her *pièce de résistance*. The grating needs to be done on the biggest hole of the grater to prevent the whole event turning to mush; take your time, it makes for a contemplative moment in a busy day. Beetroot stems and leaves can, by the way, be eaten too, so don't chuck them. Save for another salad, or sauté in garlic and olive oil until just wilted – then sprinkle with Parmesan and crack out the black pepper.

Serves four

For the salad:
3 carrots, peeled and roughly grated
½ celeriac, mandolined
3 medium raw beetroot, scrubbed and
   roughly grated
1 apple, grated and squeezed with lemon
   to prevent discolouration

For the dressing
1 tbsp horseradish sauce
1 tbsp good olive oil
1 tbsp freshly squeezed orange juice
1 tsp English mustard
1 garlic clove, peeled and crushed
salt and pepper

For the garnish:
1 tsp cumin seeds, whole or dry-roasted
   and ground
1 tbsp pumpkin seeds
coriander leaves

Assemble the grated veggies in a bowl. Combine the dressing ingredients, add to the bowl and mix well. Serve scattered with seeds and coriander leaves.

NB

SCIENTIFIC STUDIES SHOW THAT BEETROOT CAN HELP TO LOWER BLOOD PRESSURE [35]

PEA, PRAWN AND PEA SHOOT SALAD

CALORIE COUNT: **152**

This is a wonderful spring-time salad – pale green, pretty pink and dancing with clean, fresh flavours. Glitz it up with freshly podded peas and whole shell-on prawns if you are in the market for a bit of posh.

Serves two

For the salad:
100g cooked prawns, shelled
100g peas, frozen or fresh from the
    pod, just cooked
1 baby gem lettuce, washed and torn
50g pea shoots
1 spring onion, finely sliced
15g/1½ tbsps fresh tarragon, picked
handful of mint leaves

For the dressing:
1 tbsp good olive oil
1 tsp white wine or
    tarragon vinegar
½ tsp Dijon mustard
salt and pepper

Whisk dressing ingredients (you can quadruple the quantities and keep the remaining dressing in the fridge for 3-4 days). Assemble the salad ingredients, drizzle with the dressing. Toss and serve.

NB

A PORTION OF THIS SALAD DELIVERS THE SAME AMOUNT OF IRON AS A SMALL STEAK, AND THE VITAMIN C WILL AID ITS ABSORPTION

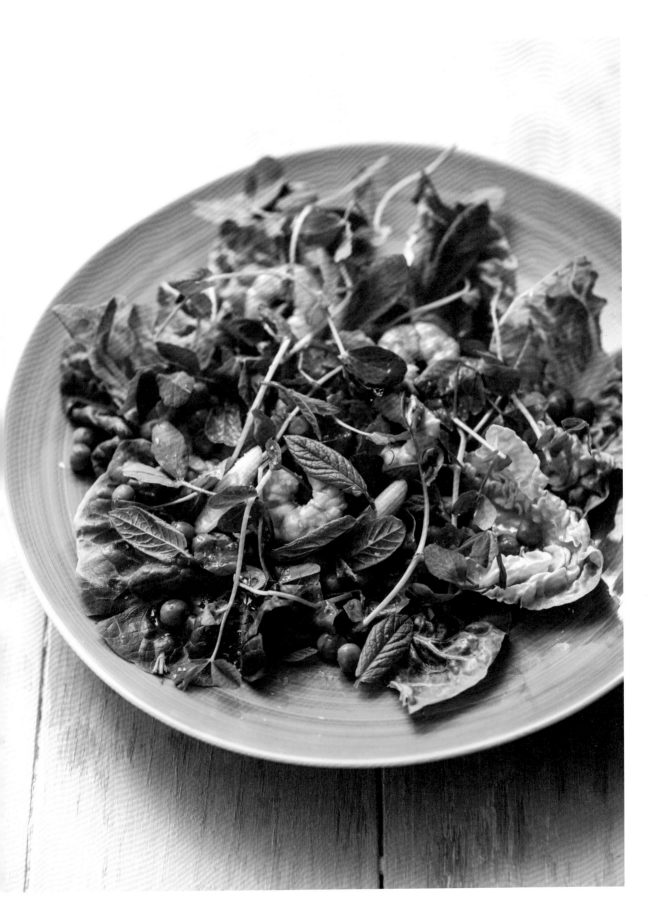

SPROUTS

CALORIE COUNT: 161

Historically, sprouts have had something of an image problem in the UK, which is an almighty shame as they are glorious little things, full of protein and unexpected flavour. There are countless varieties – broccoli, alfalfa, clover, lentil, mustard, onion, mung, soy – but I'm particularly fond of radish sprouts, which have the pepper punch of radishes and look immensely appealing on the plate, a crazy tangle of filigree filaments to confuse your fork.

Serves four

For the dressing and garnish:
1 tbsp lime juice
handful of coriander, finely chopped
1 tsp flaxseed oil
1 tsp sesame oil
½ tsp soy sauce
1 tsp root ginger, grated
1 tsp clear honey
salt and pepper
50g sunflower seeds

For the salad:
2 carrots, julienned
1 celery stalk, julienned
2 red-skinned dessert apples, cored and
   thinly sliced, squeezed with lemon
   to prevent discolouration
200g mung bean sprouts
150g alfalfa sprouts
100g radish sprouts, if available

Combine dressing ingredients, remembering that the quantities are just a guideline. Assemble the salad vegetables, dress, and scatter with seeds.

NB

PLENTY OF VITAMIN E AND A DECENT AMOUNT OF MAGNESIUM IN THIS SUPER-HEALTHY SALAD

SUPERFOOD BELLY BUSTER

CALORIE COUNT: 173

Much has been written about the towering promise of 'superfoods' – and while they do tend to offer substantial nutritional advantage, there's also a bit of marketing puff in the mix. This salad brings together an all-star cast that delivers ample vitamins, minerals and fibre with very little hype.

Serves four

For the salad:
3 tbsps quinoa, simmered for 10-12 minutes, stirred and cooled
100g broccoli florets, stem included and sliced, blanched for 2-3 minutes, drained and refreshed in cold water
100g green beans, cut into 3cm lengths, also blanched and refreshed
100g frozen peas, just cooked
100g rocket leaves
100g young spinach leaves
½ red onion, finely sliced
3 ripe tomatoes, roughly chopped
½ peeled cucumber, deseeded and sliced into crescents
handful of alfalfa sprouts

For the dressing:
juice of a lemon
1 tbsp good olive oil
salt and pepper

For the garnish:
plenty of mint and flat-leaf parsley, chopped
lemon wedges
1 tbsp sesame and pumpkin seeds, lightly toasted
pomegranate seeds

Mix the cooled quinoa with the rest of the salad ingredients. Dress with lemon and olive oil, and season. Serve the salad with chopped herbs, lemon wedges and a scatter of sesame, pumpkin and pomegranate seeds. To make a more substantial meal, add a handful of crumbled feta (add 125 calories for 50g feta).

NB

QUINOA CONTAINS DOUBLE THE PROTEIN AND MAGNESIUM, 3 TIMES THE POTASSIUM AND ZINC AND 7 TIMES THE IRON AND CALCIUM OF OTHER GRAINS SUCH AS BROWN RICE

GREEK SALAD WITH OREGANO AND MINT

CALORIE COUNT: 229

If you want to eat dairy protein on a Fast Day, feta – traditionally made from sheep's or goat's milk – is a good choice as it's lower in calories than many other cheeses. It's strongly flavoured too, so you don't need much to make its presence felt. It's worth going easy, in any case, as feta is relatively high in salt. To make the very best Greek salad, use the finest tomatoes you can find. I generally buy mine on the vine and ripen them on a sunny windowsill until they're bursting with flavour. A rock-hard, fridge-cold, anaemic tomato from a plastic tray isn't even in the same ballpark.

Serves four

For the dressing:
2 tbsps good olive oil
2 tbsps red wine vinegar
pinch of caster sugar
juice of a lemon
handful each of mint leaves and
    flat-leaf parsley, chopped
1 tsp dried oregano
salt and pepper

For the salad:
400g best-quality ripe tomatoes, quartered
    and cored
1 red onion, sliced
1 cucumber, peeled and cut into chunks
I small cos lettuce, leaves torn
12 Kalamata olives
200g good-quality feta cheese, broken into pieces

To serve:
2 wholemeal pitta breads, toasted and cut into
    fingers

Whisk together the dressing ingredients. Assemble salad, dress, and serve with hot pitta fingers.

Or try this Eastern feta salad for four, with 200g young spinach leaves, 4 ripe tomatoes, 1 tbsp toasted pine nuts and 200g feta cheese. Dress with 2 tbsps olive oil, fresh oregano, the juice of a lemon, 1 tbsp red wine vinegar, a hint of garlic, salt and pepper and a generous sprinkle of sumac, plus shards of 2 crisp toasted pitta bread (312 calories).

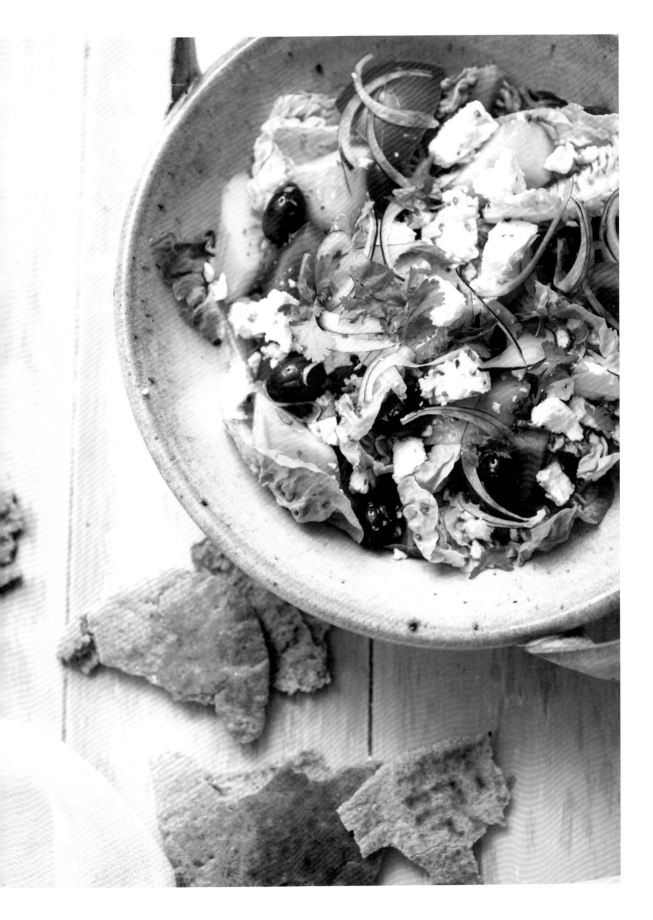

SIMPLE HERB SALAD WITH WARM BUTTERED ALMONDS

CALORIE COUNT: **236**

Fine ingredients will deliver deliciousness without too much effort, and this simple, simple salad of baby herb leaves, in season and iced, is indeed a wonderful thing. Here, a nugget of unsalted butter is, to my mind, a worthwhile calorie cost – though you could simply add the rough-chopped almonds without the need to sauté.

Serves four as a side dish

110g whole almonds, skin on
20g unsalted butter
rock salt and cracked black pepper
50g rocket
100g fresh coriander leaves, flat-leaf parsley,
    dill and tarragon, gently washed in ice-cold
    water and drained on kitchen roll
juice of a lemon
1 tbsp good olive oil

Lightly sauté almonds in the butter for 5 minutes with a good seasoning of salt and pepper. Remove from pan, set on kitchen roll to drain, then roughly chop. Assemble the rocket and herb leaves and toss gently with lemon and olive oil. Scatter with warm almonds and serve. Try this with harissa chicken, page 141.

NB

GET HALF YOUR RDA OF VITAMIN C WITH THIS SIMPLE SIDE DISH

WINTER WALDORF SALAD

CALORIE COUNT: **237** OR **298** WITH STILTON

Here's a take on the classic salad, first served at New York's Waldorf Astoria Hotel in 1893. This version is deliberately pink-cheeked, as if recently in from the cold. Go for red endive leaves, red-skinned apple and a quartered fig for prettiness. If you have calories to spare, add a hint of a hard blue cheese – perhaps some of the Christmas Stilton.

Serves two

For the salad:
1 head red endive
1 head green endive
1 red-skinned apple, chopped with a squeeze
  of lemon to prevent discolouration
2 celery stalks, chopped
50g walnut halves, broken
1 fresh fig, cut into quarters
a crumbling of Stilton, approx 30g (*optional*)

For the dressing:
2 tbsps low-fat natural yoghurt
1 tsp Dijon mustard
1 tbsp lemon juice
salt and pepper

Combine the dressing ingredients and drizzle over the salad.

NB

PLENTY OF HEALTHY MONOUNSATURATED FAT AND VITAMIN E IN THIS SALAD

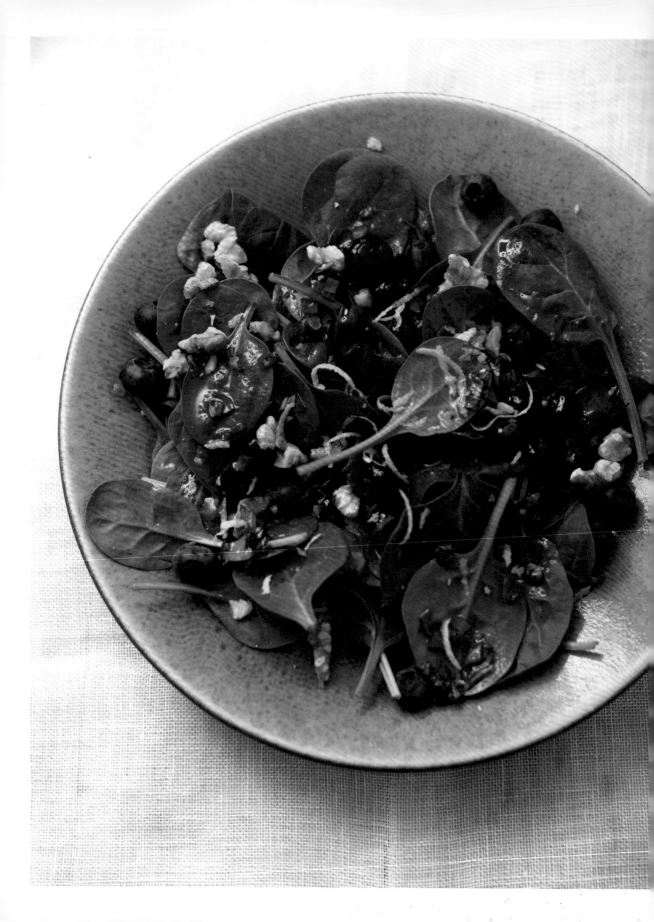

SPINACH, BLUEBERRY AND WALNUT SALAD WITH A TARRAGON VINAIGRETTE

CALORIE COUNT: **239**

I love the very idea of this salad – the pop of blueberries, the sweet tarragon, the rich crunch of walnut. It's something to chuck together on a long, hot day. No mess, no fuss, just great.

Serves two

For the vinaigrette:
2 tsps groundnut oil
2 tsps cider vinegar
zest of half a lemon
1 tbsp fresh tarragon
salt and pepper

For the salad:
200g young spinach leaves
50g walnut halves, slightly broken
100g blueberries

Prepare the vinaigrette. Then combine the spinach, walnuts and blueberries and dress. For extra bulk and texture, add 100g cooked and seasoned Puy lentils and a tangle of sautéed red onion, thinly sliced (add 159 calories).

NB

EATING BLUEBERRIES SEEMS TO OFFER NEUROPROTECTION AGAINST AGE-RELATED COGNITIVE AND MOTOR DECLINE[36]

NO-POTATO NIÇOISE

CALORIE COUNT: **253**

This is one of my favourite fall-back recipes, stacked with lots of interesting morsels and a little Riviera sophistication. If entertaining on a Fast Day – and I don't see any reason not to, as long as you can forego the goblets of wine – this makes a gorgeous glamour plate for a party. Simply multiply the quantities according to how many friends show up, and perhaps serve with griddled tuna steak rather than the tinned variety.

Serves two

1 200g tuna steak (or 160g tinned tuna in brine,
   drained which reduces calorie count by 60)
1 egg, hardboiled and plunged into cold water
salad leaves – choose soft, pretty ones like
   radicchio or lamb's lettuce
200g green beans, steamed or boiled and
   refreshed in cold water
50g cherry tomatoes, halved
8 black olives
squeeze of lemon juice
½ tbsp good olive oil
salt and pepper
2 anchovy fillets (*optional*)
lemon wedges, to serve

If using fresh tuna, season and griddle in a hot pan until cooked to your liking. Allow to rest. Assemble the leaves, cold green beans, quartered hardboiled egg, tomatoes and olives decoratively in a bowl. Dress with lemon and olive oil. Place tuna fillet or tinned tuna on top, season and garnish with anchovy fillet and lemon wedges.

NB

ONE PORTION OF THIS SALAD DELIVERS OVER 30G OF PROTEIN AND A HOST OF HEALTH-BOOSTING PHYTOCHEMICALS

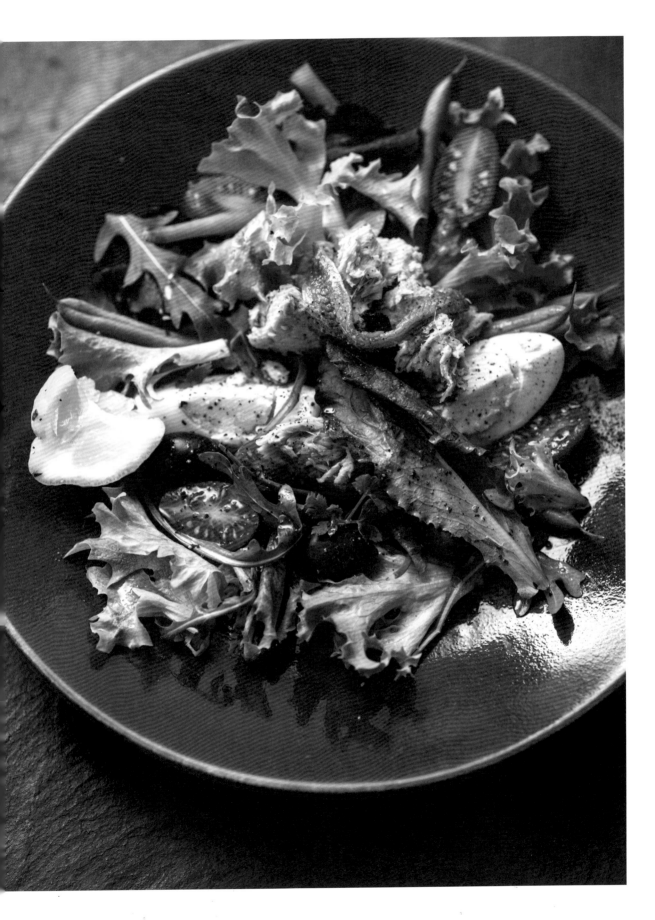

WATERCRESS, ORANGE AND ALMOND WITH A POPPY-SEED DRESSING

CALORIE COUNT: **287**

You could eat an entire kilogram of watercress for a mere 110 calories – better still, a study recently found that eating 3 ounces daily increases levels of the cancer-fighting antioxidants lutein and betacarotene.[37] OK, so that's a lot of watercress, but it does mean it's worth eating it as often as possible. I'm more entranced by its wild taste – dense, delicious and, it seems to me, the precise flavour I imagine when I think of *green*.

For the salad:
generous handful of watercress, washed
  and tough stems removed
1 orange, peeled and segmented
10 blanched almonds, roughly chopped

For the dressing:
1 tsp Dijon mustard
2 tsps red wine vinegar
½ tsp honey
2 tsps rapeseed oil
2 tsps poppy seeds
salt and pepper

Combine the salad ingredients. Drizzle with dressing and serve.

You may wish to add
- a handful of sliced chestnut mushrooms (add 5 calories)
- slivers of fennel, fennel seeds and sprigs of mint (add 3 calories)
- or swap the watercress for raw spinach or finely chopped kale, then add thin slices of red onion and 1 tsp pine nuts (add 34 calories)

NB

YOU'LL GET TWICE THE RDA FOR VITAMIN C FROM THIS SALAD – NOT A BAD THING. IF YOUR BODY NEEDS EXTRA, YOU'LL RETAIN IT; IF NOT, IT'S EXCRETED

PINK LEAVES, BLUSH FRUITS AND STILTON CRUMB

CALORIE COUNT: **333**

It's probably worth eating this salad for the title alone – but it also brings some fine Fast Day ingredients to your plate. Look for russet-skinned pears, and keep the skin on (a great source of fibre). Pears, like apples, have a relatively low GL (they score a respectable 4, about the same as a fresh fig). The suggestion of Stilton here completes the well-loved equation for the dish: pear + walnuts + blue cheese = delicious.

Serves two

1 head of endive (red makes it pretty)
handful of radicchio leaves
1 blush-skinned pear, washed, quartered, cored and
   sliced, with a squeeze of lemon to prevent discolouration
1 fig, cut into eighths
50g walnut halves
1 tbsp good balsamic vinegar
1 tbsp good olive oil
salt and pepper
pomegranate seeds to serve
50g good British Stilton, such as Cropwell Bishop or Colston Bassett

Assemble leaves in a bowl, scatter pear, fig and walnuts and dress with balsamic and olive oil. Season, then add pomegranate seeds and a snowy crumble of Stilton.

NB

PEARS ARE EASY TO DIGEST AND ONE OF THE LEAST ALLERGENIC FOODS AROUND

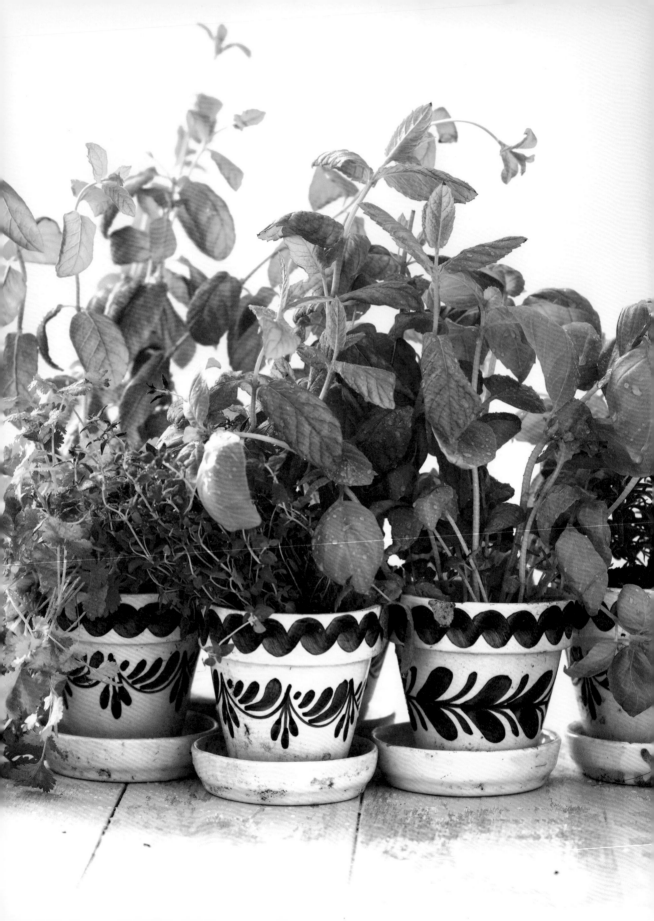

flavour saviours

Fast Day food always needs a bolt of flavour, so here are ways to add a potent boost of taste to your plate. Each recipe makes plenty, so calorie counts are for one tablespoon. The rest will keep happily in the fridge for a couple of days.

CORIANDER AND CHILLI SAUCE

CALORIE COUNT PER TBSP: 19

3 garlic cloves, peeled
1 tsp brown sugar
1 tsp galangal or root ginger, peeled
  and sliced
½ tbsp tamarind paste

2 tsps lime juice
2 tbsps water
fresh coriander leaves, chopped
1-2 fresh chillies, deseeded if you
  prefer less heat

Blitz in a processor, and serve a spoonful alongside grilled white fish.

GREEN HERB RELISH

CALORIE COUNT PER TBSP: 38

50g herb leaves (flat-leaf parsley, basil,
  mint and chives)
1½ tbsps capers, rinsed

2 garlic cloves, peeled
juice of a lemon
2 tbsps good olive oil

Blitz and serve.

SALSA FOUR WAYS

A fine way to bring a jolt of low-cal flavour to a Fast Day plate. A good salsa is all about the balance and freshness of ingredients, though it needn't rely on the classic union of tomatoes and onions. Salsa simply means sauce, so you can riff on the theme.

Classic tomato

CALORIE COUNT PER TBSP: 4

300g ripe tomatoes, skinned, deseeded and chopped
½ red onion, finely chopped
1 tbsp white wine vinegar
2 tsps lime juice
pinch of caster sugar
pinch of chilli flakes
basil leaves, torn
salt and pepper

Fennel and cucumber

CALORIE COUNT PER TBSP: 5

1 cucumber, peeled, deseeded and diced
1 fennel bulb, finely diced
½ red onion, finely diced
handful of coriander, chopped
1 tbsp white wine vinegar
1 tbsp lemon juice
salt and pepper

Watermelon

CALORIE COUNT PER TBSP: 6

200g watermelon, de-seeded and diced
2 spring onions, finely chopped
1 yellow pepper, deseeded and finely diced
handful coriander, chopped
juice of half a lime
salt and pepper

Roast tomato with chilli

CALORIE COUNT PER TBSP: 10

3 ripe tomatoes, peeled and de-seeded
1-2 whole green chillies
½ small onion, chopped
2 garlic cloves, peeled and finely chopped
¼ tsp caster sugar
rock salt and freshly ground pepper
3 tbsps chopped coriander
squeeze of lemon

Heat oven to 200°C/400°F. Bake the tomatoes, chillies and onion till just charred. When cooled, deseed the chillies and pound with garlic, sugar and rock salt. Add this mixture to the tomatoes and crush with a fork. Add coriander, lemon juice and the baked onion, and season with pepper.

CUCUMBER RAITA

CALORIE COUNT PER TBSP: 6

An Indian classic, of course, designed to calm, cool and cleanse the palate.
Do eliminate as much water as possible from the cucumber – you'll get a better
raita that way.

1 cucumber
250g natural low-fat yoghurt
fresh mint leaves, chopped
salt and pepper

Peel the cucumber and shave into long ribbons using a potato peeler. Discard the
central column of seeds. Place the cucumber strips in a colander with a scatter of
salt. Leave to stand for 10 minutes, then squeeze out excess water using kitchen
paper. Mix the ribbons with the yoghurt, stir in chopped mint leaves, season and
serve alongside any Fast Day curry.

WATERCRESS SALSA VERDE

CALORIE COUNT PER TBSP: 31

85g watercress
2 tbsps basil leaves
1 garlic clove, peeled
2 tbsps lemon juice
2 tsps olive oil

Blitz in a food processor, and serve alongside poached salmon fillets.

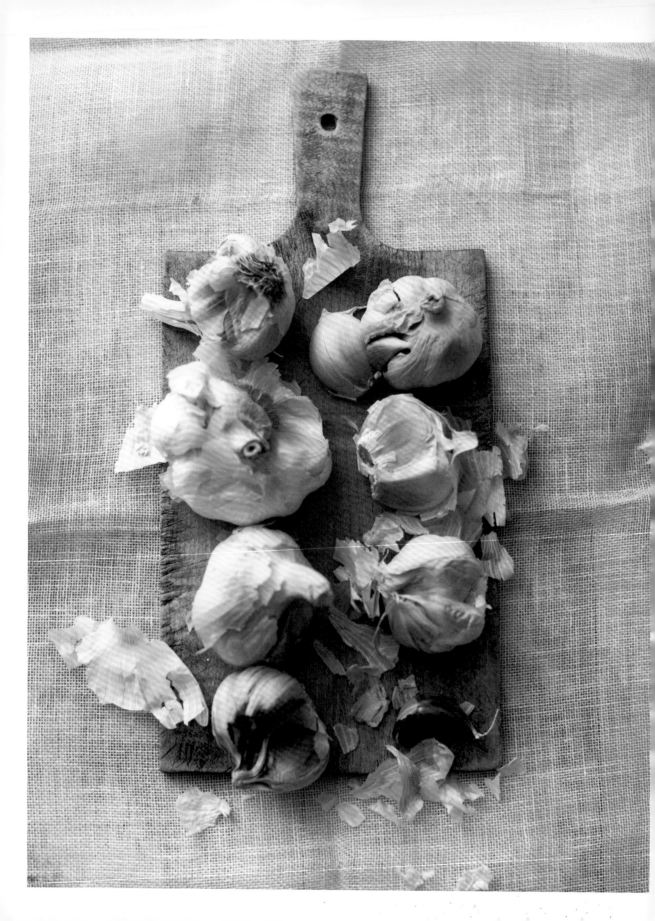

PESTO FOUR WAYS

We have come to love pesto – the classic green Italian sauce, nutty, cheesy and garlicky, is now part of the British foodscape. You can of course buy it fresh from the supermarket (avoid the jars, though – you'll be eating unnecessary preservatives). But making it is so easy. The roast red pepper pesto will save you calories, as it dispenses with cheese and nuts.

Roast pepper pesto

CALORIE COUNT PER TBSP: 12

2 garlic cloves, peeled
4 red peppers, roasted till softened and charred, seeds and stalks removed
100g basil leaves
2 tbsps good olive oil
salt and pepper

Blitz until smooth.

Parsley and pumpkin seed

CALORIE COUNT PER TBSP: 76

1 garlic clove, peeled
100g flat-leaf parsley
1 tsp sea salt
50ml good olive oil
50g pumpkin seeds

Blitz to a coarse paste.

Green classic

CALORIE COUNT PER TBSP: 71

3 handfuls fresh basil leaves
½ garlic clove, peeled
40g pine nuts
30g Parmesan, grated
1 tbsp good olive oil
1 tsp lemon juice
salt and pepper

Gently pulse the ingredients in a processor, adding a little more oil if necessary to achieve desired consistency. Serve drizzled over griddled courgette and asparagus.

Red and fiery

CALORIE COUNT PER TBSP: 90

1 garlic clove, peeled
25g pine nuts
200g semi-dried tomatoes
1 red chilli, deseeded and roughly chopped
handful of fresh flat-leaf parsley
100ml good olive oil
25g Parmesan, finely grated
salt and pepper

Pulse in a processor, keeping the paste coarse and adding a little more oil if necessary to achieve desired consistency.

THREE GOOD DRESSINGS

A salad without dressing is a marriage without love – you can get by, but no one's particularly happy. These three are well worth having in your repertoire, to be used sparingly.

Tomato vinaigrette

CALORIE COUNT PER TBSP: 13

400g ripe tomatoes, deseeded and skinned
pinch of caster sugar
2 tbsps white wine vinegar
2 tbsps good olive oil
salt and pepper

Blitz in a processor and serve with grilled fish or dark leafy salads.

Simple lemon, garlic and herb

CALORIE COUNT PER TBSP: 112

2 tbsps good olive oil
1-2 tbsps lemon juice
1 tsp Dijon mustard
1 clove garlic, peeled and crushed
salt and pepper
dried oregano or herbes de Provence

Combine and serve with grilled chicken.

Asian dressing

CALORIE COUNT PER TBSP: 22

2 tbsps soy sauce
2 tsps sesame oil
2 tsps root ginger, finely chopped
2 garlic cloves, crushed
2 tsps mirin
2 tsps lime juice
2 tbsps water

Whisk and drizzle over crisp Asian salad veggies.

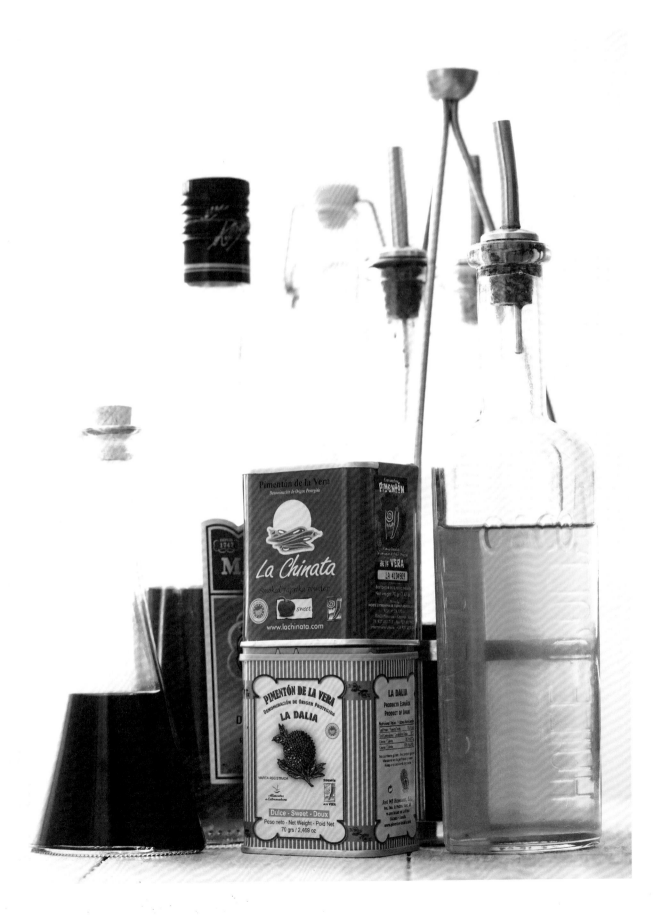

DRY RUBS

The key to brilliant Fast Day food is finding ways to impart deep, satisfying, interesting flavour without unnecessary calorie expense. While fats, oils and sugars do tend to make everything taste very good indeed (it's why we're hooked), you can easily add depth and interest without resorting to butter and cream. These dry rubs are versatile and do the job admirably, rubbed into any lean meat or fish, or sprinkled on to veggies (or how about halloumi?). Make them fresh to get maximum glory – though of course they'll keep well in an airtight jar.

Italian fennel seed and thyme

1 tbsp fennel seeds, 1 tbsp dried thyme, ½ tsp celery seeds, 1garlic clove, S&P. Pound and rub

Indian masala

½ tbsp fennel seeds, ½ tbsp coriander seeds, ½ tbsp cumin seeds, 1 tsp fenugreek, 1 cardamom pod, 1 small piece cinnamon bark, S&P, cayenne to taste. Toast in a pan. Pound and rub.

Asian

1 tbsp each of ground coriander, chilli flakes, lemongrass, ground ginger and kaffir lime leaves. Again, pound and rub.

Tunisian

1 tbsp each of garlic powder, ground cumin, ground coriander, ground ginger, paprika, turmeric, cinnamon, peppercorns. Cayenne to taste, zest of half a lemon. Pound. Rub. Good with chicken and roasted veggies.

Ras el hanout

2 tsps each of ground ginger, ground cardamom and ground mace; 1 tsp each ground cinnamon, allspice, ground coriander seeds, ground nutmeg and turmeric; ½ tsp each ground black pepper, white pepper, cayenne pepper and ¼ tsp ground cloves. Combine spices and rub well into lean steak or chicken.

Creole blackening rub

2 tsps each of pink and black peppercorns, garlic powder, smoked paprika, cayenne, sea salt, dried oregano and dried thyme; ½ tsp each of brown sugar and ground cumin; grate of nutmeg. Pound and rub.

Egyptian dukah

1 tbsp roasted hazelnuts (skins removed), 1 tbsp toasted sesame seeds, 1 tsp dry-fried coriander seeds, 1 tsp dry-fried cumin seeds, peppercorns. Pound and rub.

Texas dry rub

1 garlic clove; 2 tsps each of red peppercorns, ground cumin, mustard seeds; ½ tsp S&P, chilli powder, paprika. Pound and rub. Great with chicken.

WET RUBS

Think of these as massages and get stuck in. Most contain a little oil, but even so, they are a fine way to introduce fire and zing without too great a calorie cost.

Lemon zinger

zest and juice of a lemon, 2 tbsps olive oil, 1 garlic clove, fresh thyme, grate of nutmeg, S&P. Marinate chicken, fish or shellfish in rub, grill, and serve with plenty of lemon-dressed leaves.

North African chermoula

handful of chopped coriander, 2 garlic cloves, 1 tbsp paprika, 1½ tsps cumin, 1 tsp rock salt, ½ tsp ground ginger, cayenne to taste, pinch of saffron. Pound and mix, add 1 tbsp groundnut oil. This makes a great base for any tagine.

Jerk

2 tsps ground allspice, 1 tsp ground cinnamon, a grating of nutmeg, 3cm root ginger, peeled and finely chopped, 3 crushed garlic cloves, 2 finely chopped shallots, 1 tbsp chilli purée, 1 tbsp lime juice, 1 tbsp olive oil, handful fresh thyme leaves, S&P. Combine ingredients and rub well over a whole chicken. Roast or barbecue until cooked through.

Memphis BBQ

1 tbsp smoked paprika, ½ tbsp mustard powder, cayenne to taste, 1 tbsp maple syrup, S&P. Combine and smear on lean pork loin. Leave to marinate for an hour or more before barbecuing.

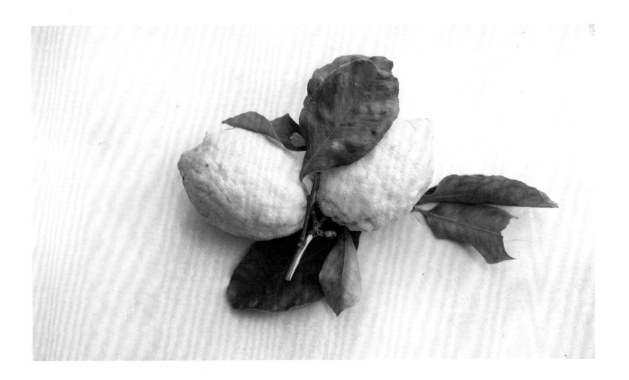

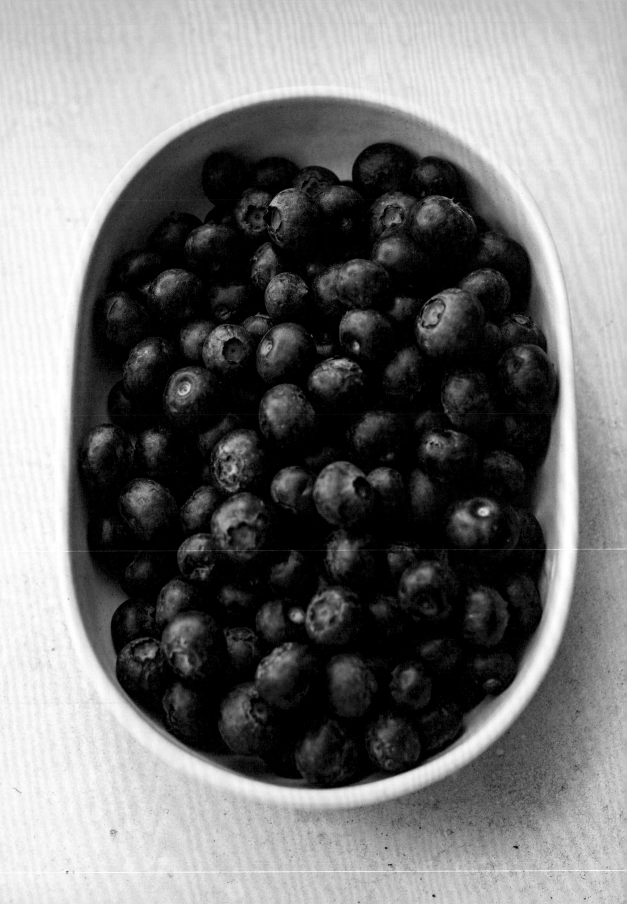

fast day snacks

There's little point in grazing on a Fast Day – it would soon eliminate the point of the exercise. But some people need a little lift, particularly in the early days when appetites are adjusting to the new regime. If tummy rumbles get the better of you, reach for one of these Super Snacks. It's best to avoid easy carbs and go instead for fresh, raw ingredients. Have them prepped and handy in the fridge. Nuts, though high in calories, are full of protein and good fats, and just a few will help you feel full.

A handful of almonds, 80 calories for 6

Crudités: carrot sticks, celery stalks, cucumber sticks, raw pepper, watercress, radishes, cherry tomatoes, approx 40 calories per serving (a medium bowlful)

A tbsp hummus, 56

Fresh strawberries, 30 calories for 10

100g blueberries, 57

60g stoned cherries, 23

100g blackberries, 25

A tbsp cottage cheese, 40

25g Edam, 85

10g air-popped popcorn, 59

Pistachios, 60 calories for 10

Apple slices, including skin and core – add a squeeze of lemon juice, 48

Plain edamame – steamed and served warm with a little rock salt, 84 calories for 60g

A medium-sized hardboiled egg, 75

A couple of hardboiled quail's eggs, 60

Pumpkin and sunflower seeds, 90 calories for 1 tbsp

A few frozen grapes, 60

Harley's sugar-free jelly pots, 4

A cup of miso soup from sachet, or a cup of hot Bovril, 32

Liquorice root to chew, 0

Something tasty or crunchy from the fridge: a bite of guindillas, pickled cucumber, sliced jalapeños or cornichons, approx 8-10 calories

meal planner

You can make up your Fast Day calories with any combination of meals – for inspiration, here's a month of plans for women and a month for men (two days for each week).

FAST 500 FOR WOMEN

	BREAKFAST	SUPPER	TOTAL CALORIES
DAY 1	Poached egg with spinach, mushroom and tomato, *page 35*	Roast sardines, *page 132*	523
DAY 2	High-energy breakfast, *page 43*	Skinny bouilllabaise, *page 177*	409**
DAY 1	Yoghurt pot with fruit, *page 30*	Lo-lo meatballs, *page 146*	528
DAY 2	Spiced pear porridge, *page 47*	Masala chicken, spinach and raita, *page 139*	505
DAY 1	Prawn omelette, *page 41*	Greek salad, *page 190*	436**
DAY 2	Strawberries with ricotta, *page 24*	Couscous with lemon tofu, *page 73*	475*
DAY 1	Eggs and asparagus, *page 23*	Tuna with chilli green beans, *page 127*	457*
DAY 2	Cherry yoghurt with muesli, *page 42*	Chicken puttanesca, *page 145*	470*

* allowance for 1 small piece of fruit or milk in tea/coffee

** allowance for an additional small snack

FAST 600 FOR MEN

	BREAKFAST	SUPPER	TOTAL CALORIES
DAY 1	Yoghurt pot with fruit, *page 30*	Hot Thai stir-fry with peanuts, *page 88*	605
DAY 2	Spinach omelette, *page 62*	Harissa chicken, *page 141*	597
DAY 1	Shakshouka, *page 36*	Griddled pheasant, *page 155*	594
DAY 2	Spiced pear porridge, *page 47*	Lightweight cottage pie, *page 142*	529**
DAY 1	Kipper and mushrooms, *page 29*	Lemon chicken and roasted veg, *page 149*	521**
DAY 2	Lean eggs (2) and ham, *page 24*	Charred chilli squid, *page 130*	547*
DAY 1	Jumbo porridge with jewel fruits, *page 32*	Tuna fagioli, *page 124*	570
DAY 2	Cherry yoghurt with muesli, *page 42*	Warming stew, *page 152*	608

RECIPES BY CALORIE COUNT

0-100 cals

100-200 cals

200-300 cals

300-400 cals

400-500 cals

Glossary

5:2 The Intermittent Fasting method devised by Dr Michael Mosley: on two days, calories are cut to a quarter of the usual intake. On the five remaining days, you eat normally

ADF Alternate Day Fasting, a version of IF, as developed by scientists including Dr Krista Varady of the University of Illinois at Chicago

CALORIE QUOTA or **BUDGET** The number of calories allowed on a Fast Day: 500 for women, 600 for men

CALORIE COST The calories in any given food

THE FAST DIET Michael and Mimi's 5:2 Intermittent Fasting method

FASTING WINDOW The number of hours between eating on a Fast Day. Aim for a 12-hour window

GI Glycaemic Index, a measure of the effect of a carbohydrate on blood sugar relative to pure glucose (which scores 100)

GL Glycaemic Load, a more useful measure which takes into account how much of the carbohydrate is in the food

$$\frac{GI \times grams\ of\ carbohydrate}{100}$$

A score of under 10 is ideal on a Fast Day

IF Intermittent Fasting: occasional periods without food, or cutting back on calories for part of the time

RDA Recommended Daily Amount, or Recommended Dietary Allowance. Also called Guideline Daily Amount or Recommended Daily Intake: the government-defined daily intake level of a nutrient considered to be sufficient for good health

Endnotes

1 Van Proeyen K, Szlufcik K, Nielens H, Pelgrim K, Deldicque L, Hesselink M, Van Veldhoven PP, Hespel P. Research Centre for Exercise and Health, Department of Biomedical Kinesiology, Leuven, Belgium. 'Training in the fasted state improves glucose tolerance during fat-rich diet'. *Journal of Physiology*, November 2010
AND
Harber MP, Konopka AR, Jemiolo B, Trappe SW, Trappe TA, Reidy PT. Human Performance Laboratory, Ball State University, Muncie, IN, US. 'Muscle protein synthesis and gene expression during recovery from aerobic exercise in the fasted and fed states'. *American Journal of Physiology*, November 2010

2 Varady, KA; Surabhi Bhutani; Church EC; Kempel, M. 'Short-term modified alternate-day fasting: a novel dietary strategy for weight loss and cardio-protection in obese adults'. *American Journal of Clinical Nutrition*, November 2009
AND
Klempel MC, Bhutani S, Fitzgibbon M, Freels S, Varady KA. Department of Kinesiology and Nutrition, University of Illinois at Chicago, IL, US. 'Dietary and physical activity adaptations to alternate day modified fasting: implications for optimal weight loss'. *Nutrition Journal*, September 2010

3 Michelle N. Harvie et al. Genesis Prevention Centre, University Hospital of South Manchester NHS Foundation Trust, UK. 'The effects of intermittent or continuous energy restriction on weight loss and metabolic disease risk markers: a randomised trial in young overweight women' *International Journal of Obesity* (London), May 2011

4 Yamamoto et al 'Therapeutic potential of inhibition of the NF- B pathway in the treatment of inflammation and cancer'. *Journal of Clinical Investigation*.
AND
Czapliska M, Czepas J, Gwodziski K; 'Structure, antioxidative and anticancer properties of flavonoids'. Postepy Biochem. 2012.
AND
Cushnie TPT, Lamb AJ. 'Recent advances in understanding the antibacterial properties of flavonoids'. *International Journal of Antimicrobial Agents*.

5 Karppi J et al, 'Serum lycopene decreases the risk of stroke in men', *Neurology* October, 2012

6 RuiHai Liu. Department of Food Science, Cornell University, New York, US. 'Thermal Processing Enhances the Nutritional Value of Tomatoes by Increasing Total Antioxidant Activity'. *Journal of Agricultural and Food Chemistry*, April 2002

7 Elizabeth E. Devore et al, 'Dietary intakes of berries and flavonoids in relation to cognitive decline', *Annals of Neurology*, July 2012

8 Mattes R. Soup and satiety. Department of Foods and Nutrition, Purdue University, 700 W State Street W. Lafayette, IN, USA. *Physiol Behav*. Jan 2005

9 M E Clegg, V Ranawana, A Shafat and C J Henry. Functional Food Centre, Oxford Brookes University, Headington, Oxford. 'Soups increase satiety through delayed gastric emptying yet increased glycaemic response.' UK *European Journal of Clinical Nutrition*, January 2013.

10 P. Schieberle, Technical University of Munich. Identifying substances that regulate satiety in oils and fats and improving low-fat foodstuffs by adding lipid compounds with a high satiety effect, 'Perception of fat content and regulating satiety: an approach to developing low-fat foodstuffs', 2009-2012

11 Pappas, AC., Karadas, F., Surai, PF., et al. (2006). 'Interspecies variation in yolk selenium among eggs of free-living birds: The effect of phylogeny.' *J Trace Elem Med Biol*, 2006

12 Dieter Schrenk, Geisenheim Research Center, Germany. 'Pectin, Fat Absorption and Anti-Carcinogenic Effects'. *Nutrition*, April 2008
AND
Lattimer JM, Haub MD Department of Human Nutrition, Kansas State University. 'Effects of dietary fiber and its components on metabolic health'. *Nutrients*, 2010

13 Dhurandhar N. Pennington Biomedical Research Center, Louisiana, US. 'Egg Proteins For Breakfast Keeps You Feeling Full For Longer'

14 RuiHai Liu. Department of Food Science, Cornell University, New York, US. 'Thermal Processing Enhances the Nutritional Value of Tomatoes by Increasing Total Antioxidant Activity'. *Journal of Agricultural and Food Chemistry*, April 2002

15 Clegg ME, Ranawana V, Shafat A, Henry CJ. Functional Food Centre, Oxford Brookes University, Headington, Oxford, UK. 'Soups increase satiety through delayed gastric emptying yet increased glycaemic response'. *European Journal of Clinical Nutrition*, January 2013

16 Meydani M, Tufts University, Boston, MA, USA. 'Potential health benefits of avenanthramides of oats'. *Nutrition Review*, December 2009

17 Aggarwal BB, Ichikawa H. The University of Texas, USA.

'Molecular targets and anticancer potential of indole-3-carbinol and its derivatives'. *Cell Cycle*, September 2005

18 Cheskin L, John Hopkins Weight Management Center. 'Lack of Energy Compensation Over Four Days when White Button Mushrooms are Substituted for Beef', *Appetite*, September 2008

19 Jenkins David J.A., MD, PhD, 'Effect of Legumes as Part of a Low Glycemic Index Diet on Glycemic Control and Cardiovascular Risk Factors in Type 2 Diabetes', *Arch Intern Med*, Nov 26, 2012

20 Stabler SN, Tejani AM, Huynh F, Fowkes C. 'Garlic for the prevention of cardiovascular morbidity and mortality in hypertensive patients'. *Cochrane Database Syst Rev.*, August 2012

21 Miglio, C; Chiavaro, E; Visconti A; Fogliano V. Department of Public Health, University of Parma, Italy. 'Effects of Different Cooking Methods on Nutritional and Physicochemical Characteristics of Selected Vegetables'. *Journal of Agricultural and Food Chemistry*, December 2007

22 Dinkova-Kostova AT, Kostov RV. 'Glucosinolates and isothiocyanates in health and disease'. *Trends Mol Med*, 2012

23 Mozaffarian D, Rimm EB. 'Fish intake, contaminants, and human health: evaluating the risks and the benefits'. *JAMA*, 2006

24 Ferreira IC, Vaz JA, Vasconcelos MH, Martins A. 'Compounds from wild mushrooms with antitumor potential. Anticancer Agents'. *Med Chem*, 2010

25 Clegg ME, Ranawana V, Shafat A, Henry CJ. Functional Food Centre, Oxford Brookes University, Headington, Oxford. 'Soups increase satiety through delayed gastric emptying yet increased glycaemic response'. *European Journal of Clinical Nutrition*, January 2013

26 Mahmoud RH, Elnour WA. 'Comparative evaluation of the efficacy of ginger and orlistat on obesity management, pancreatic lipase and liver peroxisomal catalase enzyme in male albino rats'. *Eur Rev Med Pharmacol Sci.* 2013

27 Esiyok D, Otles S, Akcicek E. 'Herbs as a food source in Turkey'. *Asian Pac J Cancer Prev.* 2004

28 Obulesu M, Dowlathabad MR, Bramhachari PV. 'Carotenoids and Alzheimer's disease: an insight into therapeutic role of retinoids in animal models'. *Neurochem Int.*, 2011

29 Vafa M, Mohammadi F. 'Effects of cinnamon consumption on glycemic status, lipid profile and body composition in type 2 diabetic patients'. *Int J Prev Med.*, 2012

30 Gazzani G, Daglia M, Papetti A. 'Food components with anticaries activity'. *Curr Opin Biotechnol.*, 2012

31 Clegg ME, Golsorkhi M, Henry CJ. Combined medium-chain triglyceride and chilli feeding increases diet-induced thermogenesis in normal-weight humans. *European Journal of Nutrition*, 2012

32 Wylie LJ, Mohr M. Dietary nitrate supplementation improves team sport-specific intense intermittent exercise performance. *European Journal of Applied Physiology*, 2013

33 Mansouri M. Tehran university of medical sciences, Tehran, Iran. The effect of 12 weeks Anethum graveolens (dill) on metabolic markers in patients with metabolic syndrome; a randomized double blind controlled trial. *Daru*, October 2012

34 Chainy GB, Manna SK, Chaturvedi MM, Aggarwal BB. Anethole blocks both early and late cellular responses transduced by tumor necrosis factor. *Oncogene,* Jun 2000
AND
Domiciano TP. State University of Maringá, Maringá, Paraná, Brazil. Inhibitory effect of anethole in nonimmune acute inflammation. Naunyn Schmiedebergs. *Arch Pharmacol.*, Dec 2012

35 Ferreira LF, Behnke BJ. 'A toast to health and performance! Beetroot juice lowers blood pressure and the O2 cost of exercise'. *Journal of Applied Physiology*, 2011

36 Devore EE, Kang JH, Breteler MM, Grodstein F. Dietary intakes of berries and flavonoids in relation to cognitive decline.

37 Gill, C, University of Ulster, Northern Ireland. 'Watercress supplementation in diet reduces lymphocyte DNA damage and alters blood antioxidant status in healthy adults'. *American Society for Clinical Nutrition*, 2007, *Ann Neurol* 2012

INDEX

Acknowledgements

My thanks to the brilliant, brilliant Rebecca Nicolson and Aurea Carpenter at Short Books, and to Katherine Stroud, Roz Hutchinson, Emmie Francis, Paul Bougourd, Catherine Gibbs, Mary J Jay, and Sallie Coolidge – the publishing dream team.

This book looks so delicious largely thanks to Romas Foord's heroic photographic sessions, along with stylist Polly Webb-Wilson and designer Georgia Vaux.

Thank you to Dr Sarah Schenker for explaining the difference between thiamin and niacin, and for counting every last calorie in the book.

My thanks to the cooks, chefs and food experts who have kindly donated recipes and good counsel to a cookbook rookie: Allegra McEvedy, Hugh Fearnley-Whittingstall, Ben McKellar, Sarah Raven and Alex Renton.

And to my friends and family, always ready with a recipe and an interesting snippet about nettles or beetroot or exactly how to poach an egg: Debbie Spencer-Jones, Julie Spencer, Claire Denholm, Marcus Fergusson and Penny Nagle. And of course to my husband and children, Paul, Lily and Ned.

Finally, thanks, as ever, to Nicola Jeal. And to Dr Michael Mosley, without whom all of this would be academic.

The authors

MIMI SPENCER has written about body shape, diet and food trends for more than 20 years – as a columnist for *Observer Food Monthly* magazine, and on *Waitrose Food Illustrated*, and as a feature writer for most national newspapers and magazines. But more than that, as she says, 'I am a mother and a wife and a cook like you, wheeling my trolley around the supermarket, desperate for inspiration about what to cook tonight. This book is as much a function of personal experience as professional know-how.' @mimispencer1

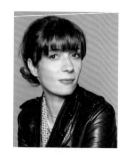

DR SARAH SCHENKER is a registered dietitian and nutritionist who has served on both professional and government committees. She now combines her sports nutrition work, consulting for football clubs including Tottenham Hotspur and Chelsea, with regular appearances on television and writing for scientific journals, as well as for newspapers, magazines and websites. Sarah is married with two young sons – so she also has a busy mum's understanding of how best to feed a family. For *The Fast Diet Recipe Book*, Sarah has used COMPEAT nutrition analysis software to complete the calorie calculations. @SarahSchenker

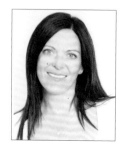